Praise for
True Wellness for Your Gut

"Hippocrates famously stated, 'All disease begins in the gut.' And, as it relates to the number-one causes of death on our planet, chronic degenerative conditions like diabetes, Alzheimer's disease, obesity, and coronary artery disease, what goes on in the gut has wide reaching and even existential implications. As such, we welcome *True Wellness for Your Gut* as it provides profoundly insightful and actionable information that may well serve to be transformative in charting the reader's health destiny."

—David Perlmutter, MD, author, New York Times
bestseller, *Grain Brain and Brain Wash*

"I recently had the pleasure of reading *True Wellness for Your Gut* and I must say I thoroughly enjoyed it. As a board-certified gastroenterologist, I found the chapters involving the anatomy and physiology of the digestive system to be very detailed and well-researched, yet concise, logically presented, and easy to understand. Not only was it an excellent review of some of the basics for me, it also allowed me to expand my knowledge in the field of gastroenterology.

"I found of particular value The Human Microbiome and Balancing the Gut-Brain-Microbiome Axis sections of chapter 3, which examine some of the most up-to-date principles of the human gut microbiota. As our knowledge of this exciting and rapidly evolving field grows, I believe it will fundamentally change how doctors and their patients approach digestive health. Furthermore, as a physician trained almost exclusively in the principles of Western medicine, I learned a great deal about how Eastern and Western medicine can complement one another. In short, without reservation I would recommend this book to anyone with a desire to improve not only their digestive well-being, but their overall health as well."

—James D. Panetta, DO, Board Certified Gastroenterologist

T0117453

"At no other time in our history has taking responsibility for our health and wellness been more imperative. Science has now shown that diet, lifestyle, and stress play an integral part in the support of our immune systems and therefore our health. Myriad health issues begin with poor dietary and lifestyle habits that lead to dysfunction of the digestive system and dysregulation of our immune function. The old adage, 'You are what you eat' rings true.

"*True Wellness for Your Gut* combines the most current discoveries of Western medicine with the ancient healing wisdom and practices of Eastern medicine to address digestive related disease. It provides an easy-to-follow guide to proper nutrition, stress management, and overall health and wellness."

—Alice Newton, National Board-Certified
Licensed Acupuncture Physician

"An informative guide to digestive health that draws on concepts from modern and traditional medicine from around the world.

"Following up on their previous book, *True Wellness: How to Combine the Best of Western and Eastern Medicine for Optimal Health* (2018), medical doctors Kurosu and Kuhn aim to bridge the gap between ancient and modern health principles in this self-help guide, which offers helpful approaches to readers struggling with digestive issues or with maintaining a healthy weight. It starts with a general overview of the philosophies behind Western and Eastern medicine (Kuhn received medical training in China and Kurosu, in North America) and then walks readers through an in-depth analysis of the human digestive system, including common digestive and metabolic illnesses such as peptic ulcers, irritable bowel syndrome, and celiac disease. After that, the chapters shift to healing methods and strategies that readers may implement on their own, such as dietary restrictions or the use of Chinese herbal supplements. The authors make it clear that they wrote the book to give sufferers clarity about the origins of their problems, but they also encourage them to reflect upon their lifestyles—and, specifically, whether they're pushing themselves too hard at work and at home, as stress can be a worsening factor. There are helpful, uncredited illustrations throughout; a chapter on qi gong practices for gut healing offers several detailed images to help readers understand its physical movements. The authors' writing style is warm and inviting, and they effectively get their points across without relying on complex jargon or a preachy tone. What's most striking about the book, however, is how it demonstrates the benefits of holistic medicine when combined with lifestyle changes and how it explains how a single aspect of digestive well-being can affect other areas of one's health.

"A valuable and wide-ranging wellness resource."

—Kirkus Reviews

CATHERINE KUROSU, MD, LAc
AIHAN KUHN, CMD, OBT

TRUE WELLNESS FOR YOUR GUT

Combine the Best of Western and
Eastern Medicine for Optimal
Digestive and Metabolic Health

YMAA Publication Center
Wolfeboro, New Hampshire

YMAA Publication Center, Inc.
PO Box 480
Wolfeboro, New Hampshire 03894
1-800-669-8892 • info@ymaa.com • www.ymaa.com

ISBN: 9781594397455 (print) • ISBN: 9781594397462 (ebook)
Cover design: Axie Breen
This book typeset in Minion Pro and Frutiger.
Illustrations by the authors unless otherwise noted.

20220707

Publisher's Cataloging in Publication

Names:	Kurosu, Catherine, author. | Kuhn, Aihan, author.
Title:	True wellness for your gut : combine the best of Western and Eastern medicine for optimal digestive and metabolic health / Catherine Kurosu, Aihan Kuhn.
Description:	Wolfeboro, New Hampshire : YMAA Publication Center, [2020] | Series: True wellness. | Includes bibliographical references and index.
Identifiers:	ISBN: 9781594397455 | 9781594397462 (ebook) | LCCN: 2020941295
Subjects:	LCSH: Gastrointestinal system--Diseases--Prevention. | Gastrointestinal system--Diseases-- Treatment. | Digestive organs--Diseases--Prevention. | Digestive organs--Diseases-- Treatment. | Metabolism--Disorders--Prevention. | Metabolism--Disorders--Treatment. | Diabetes--Prevention. | Diabetes--Treatment. | Obesity--Prevention. | Obesity--Treatment. | Self-care, Health. | Health--Alternative treatment. | Holistic medicine. | Alternative medicine. | Medicine, Chinese. | Health behavior. | Well-being. | Mind and body. | Nutrition. | Food preferences. | Exercise--Therapeutic use. | Qigong--Therapeutic use. | Meditation. | Acupuncture. | BISAC: HEALTH & FITNESS / Diseases / Gastrointestinal. | HEALTH & FITNESS / Healthy Living. | MEDICAL / Alternative & Complementary Medicine. | MEDICAL / Preventive Medicine.
Classification:	LCC: RC817 .K87 2020 | DDC: 616.3/3--dc23

NOTE TO READERS

The practices, treatments, and methods described in this book should not be used as an alternative to professional medical diagnosis or treatment. The authors and publisher of this book are NOT RESPONSIBLE in any manner whatsoever for any injury or negative effects that may occur through following the instructions and advice contained herein.

It is recommended that before beginning any treatment or exercise program, you consult your medical professional to determine whether you should undertake this course of practice.

Printed in USA.

Table of Contents

Books in the True Wellness series
True Wellness
True Wellness: The Mind
True Wellness for Your Heart
True Wellness for Your Gut

Also by Aihan Kuhn
Natural Healing with Qigong
Simple Chinese Medicine
Tai Chi in 10 Weeks

Dedicated to those who are passionate about
healing, learning, peace,
and
non-judgmental living

Foreword

GASTROINTESTINAL (GI or "gut") conditions are often seen in a general medical practice. Even though they are common, they are also potentially complex, and may be difficult to diagnose and successfully treat. Over the past few years, it has become clear that these types of problems can be well treated using a combination of Western and Eastern medical approaches. For instance, it may be found that acid reflux disease mimicking a heart problem is best treated for a short time with drugs to bring it under control, and that a life-stress situation causing the problem to begin with is better treated using meditation training, yoga, or qigong. Combining Eastern and Western medicine can be powerful, but do not make the mistake of thinking that if one form of medicine does not work, the other will. It is just not that simple. In addition, gut problems are often long-term chronic conditions associated with inflammation. You may suspect that I am saying treatment of gut issues can take time. That is quite true, since they often took some time to develop. It may also be that more than one Eastern modality may need to be combined with Western treatment. That is why this book presents several ways of addressing chronic gut conditions. I feel that *True Wellness for Your Gut* is the most important and powerful of the books making the True Wellness series. Drs. Kurosu and Kuhn have created an extremely useful modular approach to gut conditions that allows you to understand and modify treatment as you improve.

One way of viewing how Eastern and Western medicine might be combined is called the Five Rivers system. This looks at the way conditions and treatment styles can be divided into five areas. Here are some examples:

1. Those conditions best treated with Western medicine. (Severe trauma, potentially life-threatening acute disease, or a disease requiring specific medications such as in severe endocrine disorders.)
2. Those conditions best treated with Eastern medicine. (Imbalances between different organ systems not well defined by Western medical

concepts but quite clearly defined by Eastern medicine using what are called symbolic correspondences.)

3. Those conditions effectively treated with either system. (Gastric ulcer, allergies.)
4. Those conditions best treated by the two systems combined. (Certain cancers, pain syndromes.)
5. Those not well treated by either system. (Many cancers, genetic conditions.)

I consider this to be what I call a "next step" book. By this I mean you can start with whatever diagnosis you might have and work on developing your own associated treatment plan. You work with this for a while, get some results, and then want to do more. So you take the next step and learn more about your medical condition and treatment. This is the power of *True Wellness for Your Gut*. It is not a book that you read once and then put on the shelf to get dusty. It is a well-thought-out reference and plan of action. As you improve your condition, you will gain confidence in always being able to take the next step toward your true wellness. Finally, one of the most important steps you can take is to follow the True Wellness checklist, especially the encouragement to do something for fun each day. This may be more powerful than anything else you do!

Michael M. Zanoni, Ph.D., L.Ac.
Diplomate in Oriental Medicine, NCCAOM

Preface

IT IS RARE THESE DAYS to come across a person who is able to eat a wide array of foods, maintain a healthy weight, and not suffer any ill effects from what they choose to consume. Most of us know people who must restrict their diets because of problems like food sensitivities that cause gastrointestinal pain and digestive problems, problems with glucose utilization that causes diabetes, and the multifactorial dysregulation of metabolism that has led to our current obesity epidemic.

These people, our friends and family, are often confused by the disconnect between what they are told by their healthcare providers and what they are sold in supermarkets and fast food restaurants. The pseudo-foods created by the processed food industry are laden with refined sugars, salt, and poor-quality fats and lack vital nutrients. Moreover, such foods are targeted to children and play havoc with their digestion and metabolism. Pseudo-foods often contain ingredients such as corn and soy. These crops are heavily subsidized and allow purveyors of processed foods to sell them cheaply. Consumers of all economic levels are finding it more and more difficult to purchase organic whole foods not only because of the increased cost but often also limited access. In some areas, most of the available food is processed, prepackaged, and high in excess salt, sugar, and unhealthy fats.

Even if you are fortunate enough to have the income and access to buy organic produce and pastured meat, there is disagreement among researchers about what, when, and how we should eat. Which style of eating is best, vegan, vegetarian, pescatarian, or omnivore? Raw food only? Cooked food only? Should we intermittently fast? Should we eat whole grains or any grains at all? Eggs and nutritious fats that were vilified for decades are now back on the menu. It is hard to know what to do and who to trust.

Aside from our desire to choose foods that will promote longevity and well-being, there are many among us who must *avoid* certain foods that have become detrimental to our health. By trial and error, some people have discovered that their myriad symptoms, including digestive distress, weight gain, and impaired glucose metabolism, resolve when they avoid gluten, dairy, sugar, soy, eggs, grains, or any combination of these common foods. It is hard to imagine, but a supposedly healthy food may actually be killing you from the inside out. Unfortunately, many people with such problems are still searching for a solution. You may be one of these people and that is why you are reading this book.

True Wellness for Your Gut was written for you. The information in the following chapters will help you understand the underlying cause of your condition and ways you can solve your own problem with the help of your healthcare team. We encourage the incorporation of Eastern healing modalities such as acupuncture, meditation, and qigong into your conventional care and will explain the science behind these techniques. We feel this integration is vitally important to your success for the following reason: stress management.

If long rounds of testing and different dietary modifications fail to improve gastrointestinal and metabolic conditions, healthcare providers will finally advocate examining underlying physical and emotional stress as a possible cause of these problems. We feel strongly that stress management should be addressed concurrently with dietary and lifestyle strategies. There are many excellent books available that examine these issues from a predominantly Western perspective. That approach is entirely valid, and we list some of those books in our Recommended Reading and Resources section. This book examines the science that underlies both Western and Eastern modalities, which can both strongly and positively influence your body's response to chronic stress. After giving you an understanding of what may be causing your condition, we concentrate on lifestyle interventions that will help restore your health and well-being. Sometimes hard questions need to be asked and answered. Are you happy? Do you feel safe in your own home or neighborhood? Are you treated with respect by your family or in your work environment? Very often, physical or emotional abuse predates these conditions, and the earlier in life this abuse occurs, the greater the likelihood that illness will follow. Of course, we cannot forget about physical stressors such as poor sleep, shift work, overwork, and lack of exercise. Qigong, meditation, and acupuncture can facilitate your healing by decreasing stress, improving your sleep and exercises routine, and enhancing the function of your gastrointestinal system.

Many people assume that if digestive and metabolic diseases run in their families they are doomed to a similar fate. In most cases, this is simply not true. We now know from the study of advanced genetics, called epigenetics, that the way genes are expressed as physical conditions can be modified by the food you eat, the quality and quantity of your sleep, your exercise regimen—and even your thoughts! Even though the way you eat, working too much, and sleeping too little may have contributed to your health problems, the good news is that it is never too late to improve your condition if you are willing to make these positive lifestyle modifications. We have seen our patients adopt these changes and reap the benefits. We know you can too!

How to Use This Book. Eastern medicine has always been a whole-systems approach to health. So often, modifying general lifestyle behaviors will lead to improvements in a vast array of medical conditions. Gastrointestinal problems, diabetes, and obesity are prime examples of illnesses that Western medicine has had difficulty treating, even with high-tech procedures and pharmaceuticals. Failure often occurs because patients and doctors alike have such faith in cutting-edge medical advances that they think they do not need to pay attention to the root cause of an illness, and that surgery or medication alone can and will solve the problem. That may be true initially, but if no changes are made to the internal and external environment in which the illness developed, then it is very likely the illness will recur.

This is where combining Eastern and Western medicine can have the greatest impact. By all means, take advantage of the often life-saving techniques of modern science, but remember to go back to basics. *True Wellness for Your Gut* is designed to highlight and explain the importance of sleep, exercise, nutrition, and mindfulness to gastrointestinal and metabolic conditions. There is a lot of overlap in our recommendations for people with any or all of these diseases. That is the nature of the whole-systems approach of Eastern medicine and all other holistic medical practices.

Even so, there will be some differences. Not every reader will be suffering from diabetes *and* obesity *and* gastrointestinal problems. With that in mind, we wrote this book so that it could be read in a modular fashion.

Everyone with any sort of digestive or metabolic concern should read chapters 1, 2, 6, and 7.

Chapter 1 will give you a historical and philosophical overview of Eastern and Western medicine and the gastrointestinal system in particular. You will also learn about the science behind the Eastern medical modalities of meditation, qigong, and acupuncture as well as how they are integrated into healthcare in the twenty-first century.

Chapter 2 discusses the organs that make up the digestive system and how they work together to break down and metabolize your food, eliminate the leftover byproducts of this process, and how bacteria in your gastrointestinal tract influence all aspects of your health—from your weight to the strength of your immune system to your mental acuity and your mood. The dangers of chronic inflammation and the importance of restorative sleep in digestive and metabolic health will be addressed. In this chapter, you will also find a brief overview of the causes and definitions of various gastrointestinal diseases, diabetes, and obesity.

In chapter 6 you will learn more about the ancient art of qigong and receive step-by-step instructions to start your healing qigong practice.

Chapter 7 reinforces the principles of healthy living and shows you how to use the "True Wellness Checklist" to achieve your goals.

Integrative treatment strategies specifically for gastrointestinal diseases, diabetes, and obesity will be addressed in chapters 3, 4, and 5, respectively. You can tailor your reading to fit your health concerns. Some readers may need to read all three of these chapters. There will be some different recommendations for each condition, but because dysregulation of the digestive system and metabolism are so intimately connected, some foundational information is repeated. So if you are reading only one or two of the three chapters of treatment approaches, you will still have all the information you need to embark on your healing journey. We hope you will be patient with us when we repeatedly, but gently, remind you to apply these tried-and-true foundational healing behaviors to your daily life: sleep adequately, breathe deeply, eat nutritiously, move mindfully, and ensure that you make time for a pursuit that brings you joy.

Wishing you every success on your road to optimal health.

Aihan Kuhn, CMD, OBT
Catherine Kurosu, MD, LAc

CHAPTER 1

The Gut—An East-West Perspective

FROM THE ANCIENT to the modern world, Mother Earth has provided an abundance of food to keep us alive and give us energy for work and leisure. Our concept of the ways in which food is transformed into energy has changed over the millennia, and our understanding of the mechanism of digestion and metabolism is being continuously refined. In fact, we have come to appreciate that the gastrointestinal system is not just a conglomerate of organs that extracts nutrients from food to fuel physiologic processes. It is a complex, symbiotic web of human cells and trillions of microbes that together influence the physical and emotional health of your entire body. This intricate human-microbe relationship is known as the human microbiome, and we will take a much closer look at it throughout this book. Now let's trace the development of our understanding of the gut.

A Brief History of the Gut

Even before conscious thought, the need to eat was a biological imperative. Through trial and error, humans, like animals, discovered which plants or other creatures could be consumed without risk of illness or death. Over time, people observed that when they ate certain fruits, roots, herbs, or animals, they experienced reproducible outcomes; one root would cause diarrhea, another would relieve abdominal pain. This flower would make a person sleepy, that one would make them agitated. From these observations, the concept of food as medicine arose, but it was the keen day-to-day attention to food procurement, preparation, ingestion, and digestion that kept people healthy.

In all ancient cultures there were rules and recommendations about food as well as theories about how food was transformed into the essence that nourished life. Healers from all parts of the earth recognized a spiritual, even magical, aspect to the digestive process. In modern times we tend to take eating for granted; not only the ease with which some societies obtain food, but the innate capacity of the body to convert plants and animal meat into energy for living. Every year, medical researchers unveil more of the mysteries of the gastrointestinal system, but millennia ago the digestive process was mere conjecture.

Theories of digestion in several ancient medical systems were similar in some respects. Early Indian, Chinese, and Greek physicians all thought that whatever was present in the universe was present in the body. Therefore, they thought, food was composed of, and created by, all the building blocks of the natural world. From a technical viewpoint, food must be ingested, chewed thoroughly, and swallowed. Once it arrived in the stomach, it was subjected to some sort of heating process that caused the food to change into a substance that could more readily be used by the body. In India, Ayurvedic healers called this biological fire "agni."[1] The ancient Greeks had a similar concept of biological fire that they called "ignis." The Chinese, as we shall see, also describe an internal fire essential for digestion. According to the thinking of all these cultures, this process must be balanced or disease will result.

Ancient Greek physicians taught that digestion began in the stomach where food was changed into a substance called "chyme." Chyme is still the term we use today to describe food that has been processed and broken down in the stomach, yielding a partially digested slurry. After food was changed into chyme, it was thought to be transformed into the four components the Greeks called "humors." These are blood, mucus (or phlegm), bile, and black bile. The humors were considered the agents of metabolism—the building blocks that nourish the body and contribute to its growth and function. The humors were said to move through four stages of digestion, beginning from the stomach to the liver, then through the blood vessels to the organs, and lastly to the tissues. Although not

---

1. B. Ravishankar and V. J. Shukla, "Indian Systems of Medicine: A Brief Profile," *African Journal of Traditional Complementary and Alternative Medicine* 4 no. 3 (Feb 2007): 319–337, https://doi.org/10.4314/ajtcam.v4i3.31226.

physiologically correct, this system shares some similarities to the way food actually is digested to nourish all the cells of the body.

In China, the warming energy of the key organs of digestion (Spleen and Stomach[2]) was compared to the fire under a cauldron that cooks food. The Spleen and Stomach are said to harvest the component within food that supports life. This is called "qi." For historical and pragmatic reasons that we will discuss later, qi is often compared to the Western concept of energy. This comparison is too simplistic. It is important to note that qi is more dynamic than substantive and quantifiable. It is better understood as the transformation that occurs within an event or process.[3] In Eastern medicine, there are various subtypes of qi, each with its own function. All the other organ systems are dependent upon the qi that the Spleen and Stomach extract from the food, so if this system is disturbed, the entire body suffers. The pre-eminence of the digestive system is a feature of all medical systems and is founded on the obvious truth that deficient digestion leads to disease.

The Spleen and Stomach, together known as the Middle Jiao or Middle Burner, are responsible for all functional aspects of the organs of the gastrointestinal tract, including the transportation of nutrients throughout the body. This paradigm has similarities to and differences from what we know about the digestive system in Western medicine. As in Western medicine, digestion begins in the mouth where the food is chewed, breaking it into smaller pieces. In the Stomach, the food is separated into qi and waste products. The qi is considered to be a pure extract of the food. The Stomach is also responsible for moving waste products further down the digestive tract. From the Spleen, the qi from the food is sent to the Lungs where it combines with the qi of the air. This mixture is then further distilled into several subtypes of qi that are distributed by the Spleen to all the other organs and tissues of the body. This process is known as "transformation and transportation" or "digestion and distribution."[4]

---

2. To avoid confusion, throughout this book the names of the functional organ systems recognized by Eastern medicine are capitalized and the names of the organs from Western anatomy are lowercased.

3. Stephen J. Birch and Robert L. Felt, *Understanding Acupuncture* (Edinburgh: Churchill Livingstone, 1999), 121.

4. Will Maclean and Jane Lyttleton, *Clinical Handbook of Internal Medicine*, Volume 2: Spleen and Stomach (Sydney: University of Western Sydney, 2002), xvii.

In Eastern medicine, the Liver has a very strong influence over the Spleen and Stomach in an energetic sense. The Liver is responsible for the harmonious movement of qi throughout the body. The dyad of the Spleen/ Stomach and the Liver is central to the supply and effortless dissemination of qi. Later in this chapter we will discuss how the qi of the organs influence each other. The Small and Large Intestines serve to shepherd the waste products out of the body. In Western medicine, the functions of the small and large intestines are distinct. Ancient practitioners of Eastern medicine did not have the technology to determine the biochemical functions of the intestines. Also, the function of the pancreas was unknown at that time. We now know how essential the pancreas is to digestion and metabolism. So, in the absence of modern investigative techniques, the enzymatic, hormonal, and neurological contributions of the intestines and pancreas were described as the "transformation" of food and were attributed to the Spleen and Stomach. These observations and associations were established more than two millennia ago and have been used for thousands of years in the diagnosis and treatment of digestive and metabolic diseases.

In the West, various theories regarding digestive function were put forward over the centuries. Building upon the explanations of ancient Greek physicians, Galen (c. 130–200 CE) added the ideas that blood level was proportional to food intake and that processes in the intestines brewed food into body fluids. These theories held for more than 1,300 years until Andreas Vesalius (1514–1564) published correct anatomic descriptions of the human digestive tract, based on autopsies. With the advent of the light microscope about one hundred years later, the anatomy of the gastrointestinal tract was further clarified, even to the cellular level.

Of course, knowing the form of an organ does not automatically reveal its function. It turns out that Galen was on the right track when he proposed that food gets brewed into other bodily substances. In the 1600s, starting with the Flemish physician and chemist, Jan Baptiste van Helmont (1579–1644), various researchers added to our knowledge of the function of the digestive system and its biochemical processes. By the middle of that century, it became known that saliva had digestive ability, the stomach contained acidic fluids, and the intestinal fluids were alkaline. Diseases of the digestive system were then understood as imbalances between acid and alkali. Investigations into the function of the pancreas and the gallbladder had also begun, though the discovery and isolation of insulin from pancreatic cells would not happen until 1921.

In Italy, Lazzaro Spallanzani (1729–1799) demonstrated that the stomach produces substances other than acid that digest food. He conducted an experiment in which he had people swallow a small sponge that was tied to a thread. After retrieving the sponge, Spallanzani squeezed out the stomach juices from the sponge and applied them to both meat and a flower. The meat began to dissolve, but the flower did not. This indicated that there was more to stomach juice than acid.[5]

Across the Atlantic, more discoveries were to be made. In 1822, William Beaumont, an army physician, was stationed at Fort Mackinac in the territory of Michigan. This fort and nearby trading post were situated on the northern peninsula that separates Lake Huron and Lake Michigan. It was a center of commerce in the summer months when French Canadian and Indian trappers employed by the American Fur Company would bring in the furs from animals they had caught over the winter.

In June of that year, Dr. Beaumont was summoned to attend to a young French Canadian man named Alexis St. Martin who had been accidentally shot in the stomach. Dr. Beaumont found that not only had St. Martin's stomach been injured, a portion of his lung was protruding from the wound. Even though St. Martin was not expected to survive, Dr. Beaumont tended his injuries. Incredibly, the young man lived, but was debilitated and unable to work. The gunshot wound had healed, but in an unusual fashion. The stomach wall and abdominal wall had not healed closed in layers, but rather only the edges of the wound healed. The edges of the stomach wound had stuck to the edges of the damaged muscle and skin. This left St. Martin with a hole about the circumference of a finger that connected the inside of his stomach with the outside skin of his abdomen. In medical terms, this is called a gastrocutaneous fistula.

Dr. Beaumont took St. Martin into his home and supported him. Over time, he made notes of his observations of the fluid that was frequently emitted from the stomach fistula. From 1825 to 1833, Beaumont conducted

---

5. A. Skrodka, "A Short History of Gastroenterology," *Journal of Physiology and Pharmacology* 54, S3 (2003), 9–21.

many experiments with this fluid and observed how it was involved in the digestion of food, both outside and inside of St. Martin's stomach. These investigations were published in 1833. *Experiments and Observations on the Gastric Juice and the Physiology of Digestion* was a 280-page book containing general comments about gastrointestinal conditions and descriptions and inferences of 238 experiments conducted over eight years.[6]

In an essay published in 1902, the renowned physician Dr. William Osler summarized Beaumont's contributions to the study of gastroenterology as follows:[7]

- Accurately and completely describing gastric juice
- Confirming that hydrochloric acid was an important component of gastric juice
- Recognizing that gastric fluid and mucus were separate entities
- Establishing the influence of a disturbed mental state on the secretion of gastric juice and digestion in general
- Comparing the actions of gastric fluid inside and outside of the stomach
- Presenting the first comprehensive study of the movements of the stomach
- Creating a table of the digestibility of various foods

Thousands of years before William Beaumont and Alexis St. Martin, traditional healing systems acknowledged the link between emotions and the digestive and metabolic systems. Physicians from earlier times knew through observation that interaction between the emotions and the physical body was bidirectional, each affecting the other. Modern Western medicine used to look at the gut as strictly a mechanical and biochemical machine that would process food and absorb its nutrients—that is, until now. Over recent decades, stunning discoveries have come to light about the ways that our digestive and metabolic systems interact with our immune, hormonal, and nervous systems and echo the observations of our ancestors.

---

6. Charles Steward Roberts, "William Beaumont, the Man and the Opportunity," in *Clinical Methods: The History, Physical, and Laboratory Examinations,* third edition, ed. H. K. Walker, W. D. Hall, and J. W. Hurst (Boston: Butterworths, 1990), https://www.ncbi.nlm.nih.gov/books/NBK459/.

7. Roberts, "William Beaumont, the Man and the Opportunity."

But there is one discovery that no one could have imagined—the finding that there are trillions of microbes living within us that are indispensable to our physical and emotional well-being. These microbes have been dubbed "the human microbiome." We are only just beginning to understand the ways in which we are interconnected. In the following chapters we will describe the microbiome in depth and how it is integral to our digestive and metabolic health.

We will also discuss the ways in which you can integrate the cutting-edge science of the West and the ancient wisdom of the East into your quest for optimal digestion and metabolism. To combine these modalities for the greatest advantage we feel that an understanding of the history and philosophy of both healing systems is essential. We devote the next two sections to this topic. We will also discuss the science behind the Eastern healing arts and how your Western healthcare provider can incorporate Eastern medicine into your care. Once this groundwork has been laid, we will delve into the intricacies of the gastrointestinal system and the human microbiome, how their interaction influences your digestion and metabolism, and how integrating Western and Eastern modalities can lead to optimal health.

The History and Philosophy of Western Medicine

Hippocrates is considered the father of Western medicine. He felt that a clear understanding of the patient's way of life and constitution was essential to provide appropriate medical care. He particularly emphasized balance in daily living regarding food and exercise. As mentioned earlier, in ancient Greece, the human body was thought to be composed of material substances called "humors": blood, phlegm, bile, and black bile. Additionally, the humors were associated with certain qualities (hot, cold, moist, and dry) and elements (earth, air, fire, and water). Perfect health was considered to be the ideal equilibrium of the humors, qualities, and elements within each individual, and disease was the result of imbalances among these components.

Even prior to the birth of Hippocrates, Greek philosophers and physicians were fascinated with the natural world and, like the Chinese, used observations of their environment to explain human growth and development. It was thought that the universe consisted of pairs of opposite qualities such as hot and cold, moist and dry. Harmony between these pairs was considered paramount as an imbalance could result in disease. This principle of paired opposites is also seen in the Chinese theory of yin and yang, which we will discuss shortly.

In Europe through the Renaissance and into the Scientific Revolution (1450–1630 CE), doctors were able to use advancing technology to examine the intricate workings of the human body and their environment. For example, in 1609 the light microscope was invented and for the first time doctors and scientists could see organisms invisible to the naked eye. They called such organisms microbes. Over the next two centuries, an understanding of these organisms developed. It was proven that microbes, further classified as bacteria, viruses, and molds, could cause disease. Once it was known that specific organisms caused specific diseases, treatments were created that could cure many illnesses that had previously resulted in severe disability or death. Over time, vaccines were invented that could prevent some diseases altogether. The study of microbiology and the development of antibiotics and vaccines are some of the most significant discoveries of Western medicine.

With this astounding success in the treatment of infectious disease, Western physicians realized that if they could find the cause of an illness, they might be able to develop a cure. From this point onward, the study of medicine focused on the search for the simplest single explanation for the origin of a whole host of ailments. The Industrial Revolution in Europe was in full swing, and the study of medicine was influenced greatly by the societal changes of this era. Factories emerged, and every part of the production process was compartmentalized. No longer did an artisan see the creation of an item through from start to finish. Rather, a worker manufactured one portion of the item, then passed it on to the next worker and then the next, until completion. This fragmentation became pervasive in Western medicine too. Technology gave physicians and scientists the ability to break down biochemical and physiological processes into ever-smaller component parts; this has led to an unprecedented understanding of the complexity of the human body.

New discoveries are still being made: from the understanding that a person's constitution can be passed down to offspring to the complete mapping of the human genome, and from realizing that living things are made up of cells to understanding how these cells function and how we can use modern medicine to change these processes.

One of the main difficulties of this explosion of knowledge is how to master it and implement it correctly. As mentioned, the production line increased efficiency during the Industrial Revolution, with each worker perfecting a certain aspect in the manufacturing process. Modern medicine has also undergone a similar division of labor. With the increasing complexity of biomedicine, it has become impossible to know everything about the human body: how we get sick, how we heal, and all the possible therapeutic interventions that can be used for every illness. Medical students the world over gain basic knowledge in anatomy, physiology, and biochemistry, then branch out to learn about the many causes of disease and how to cure or improve a patient's condition. Upon graduating from medical school, young doctors in most countries are required to train further. They choose from many branches of medicine and become specialists in that field. Even those doctors who want to become family physicians do a three-year residency in general medicine to hone their skills. Others choose among general surgery, internal medicine, obstetrics and gynecology, psychiatry, radiology, or pathology. After completing at least four years in their specialty, they can then subspecialize—they can focus on the medical or surgical aspects of any single body part or process. From the brain to the feet and everything in between, you can find a subspecialist to meet your needs.

But even as a subspecialist, it is difficult to keep up with every new scientific discovery in the field. Subdividing and specializing medical research and care is a way of trying to achieve this impossible task. Similarly, the search for the single underlying cause of a particular disease is a way for modern medicine to develop treatments that hope to correct problems at the cellular, genetic, or molecular level of the body. In many instances, this approach has been spectacularly successful. For example, the discovery of the underlying cause of type-1 diabetes led to the discovery of insulin and methods for isolating it from animal sources. We are now able to manufacture insulin synthetically. Furthermore, we can even transplant the cells that create insulin, allowing diabetics to survive. Without the curiosity and ingenuity of physicians and scientists, this and other medical breakthroughs would not have been possible.

For many conditions, however, this reductionist approach has not been successful or has even created more problems. The biomedical model of seeking out a solitary cause for an illness may overlook the possibility of interplay among many factors that can contribute to a disease. These factors can be specific to an individual, like genetics, family environment, and personal life experience, or they can be factors that affect the community at large, like environmental pollution, food additives, and poor access to markets with fresh produce or green spaces in which to exercise.

The dynamics of the origins of disease are highly complex, especially with respect to the chronic diseases of Western societies, such as heart disease, type-2 diabetes, autoimmune conditions, and some gastrointestinal disorders. For many of these conditions, the biomedical model may not be the best way to institute effective health care. A growing body of evidence suggests that optimizing the way we eat, move, think, and sleep can do more to reverse chronic illness than medications or surgery. Adopting such lifestyle changes may even help to prevent these conditions in the first place.

With the realization that so many of our modern-day illnesses stem from being sleep-deprived, overfed, under-exercised, and stressed, the philosophy of Western medicine is coming full circle. We are returning to the idea that physicians must consider all aspects of a person and that person's illness, just as Hippocrates did. In this patient-centered model, the emotional, spiritual, psychological, and socioeconomic factors involved are examined alongside the physical aspects of a disease. This understanding, rooted in the origins of Western medicine, can help medical providers guide patients toward optimal health and healing.

The History and Philosophy of Eastern Medicine

Before discussing the chronology of Eastern medicine, an appreciation of its philosophy is extremely important. The principles of Eastern medicine hinge on the concept that man is inseparable from the universe. This no-tion comes from the observations and practices of Daoism. Daoism is a philosophical system that was reportedly founded by Laozi (b. 604 BCE). Although Laozi formulated the tenets of Daoism, it was his students and followers who wrote the majority of the formal texts that are the foundation of this philosophy. Prior to the advent of Daoism in China, as in every primitive civilization, the ancients observed the changes that took place over time in the world around them. They noted the cycles of the moon, planets, and stars. These celestial patterns were correlated with weather changes, growing seasons, and animal migrations. Daoism grew out of this naturalist school of thought as it attempted to understand man's place in the order of the universe. This law of nature is called the Dao. In English, this translates to "the Way" or "the Path." The Dao represents the basic principles from which all phenomena follow, including all aspects of human behavior.

In addition to the ideas of the Dao and the phases in the physical world that change over time, Daoist thinkers helped formalize the concept of the unity of opposites within nature. This is the basis of yin-yang theory for which Eastern medicine is known. By starting with the concept of opposition to describe the relationship between two entities, Daoists formulated a dynamic view of the world that could be used to explain universal processes. A classic example of this mode of thought is the observation that there is always a sunny side and a shady side to a hill. Everything can be seen as either yin or yang depending on its degree of substantiality. If something is more passive and receptive in nature, it is yin. If it is more active and dynamic, it is yang. But these definitions have meaning only when compared to one another. Any of the pairs that embody yin and yang cannot be separated and are not absolute. Moreover, while all phenomena contain both yin and yang aspects, they are not necessarily represented in equal parts. The balance must be appropriate for each unique entity or circumstance.

The yin-yang experience is a fundamental factor in the development of the Daoist philosophy. Far from designating yang as "something" and yin as "nothing," Daoism recognizes that both are active and that one creates the other.[8] For example, the ceramic of a teacup would be considered

---

8. Michael M. Zanoni, PhD, conversation with author (CK), April 10, 2011.

yang and the space within the teacup considered yin. It is the space that is filled, and therefore makes the ceramic useful as a teacup. The yin and the yang of the cup are inseparable.

From this thought arises the realization that the part and the whole must exist simultaneously. The infinite exists at every singular point in space, and eternity is found in every individual moment. The Daoist consideration of the infinite and the yin-yang experience infuse themselves into the practice of Eastern medicine by virtue of the fact that dysfunction within patients, known as the pattern of disharmony, cannot be viewed separately from the patients themselves. The part and whole exist together and define each other.

In addition to the concepts of Dao and yin-yang, the recognition of the phases of the universe was developed into the theory known as Wu Xing, or Five Phases. Wu Xing has also been translated as Five Elements; however, many scholars state that this characterization is incorrect. The word "element" implies a component part or constituent ingredient; the word "phase" denotes a dynamic process. In his iconic book, *The Web That Has No Weaver*, Dr. Ted Kaptchuk describes the Five Phases as patterns that occur in dynamic systems. Each phase has a designated name and displays a set of particular characteristics.[9] The phases are known as Wood, Fire, Earth, Metal, and Water. The names of the phases are not as important as each set of characteristic qualities and functions. Wood represents growth. Fire represents maximal growth that has reached its apex and will plateau or decline. Metal is emblematic of decline. Water denotes a profound state of rest that has reached its nadir and will shift toward growth or activity. Earth represents balance.[10] If you imagine a pendulum swinging to and fro, the Earth Phase would be the moment at which the pendulum is hanging straight down. The patterns of the Five Phases can be seen in the ebb and flow of all natural and even man-made phenomena: human growth, maturation, and decline; the changing of the seasons; economic expansion and recession; the rise and fall of political powers. In both Eastern and Western medicine, the functional systems of the body experience this ebb and flow as constant self-regulation to maintain

---

9. Ted J. Kaptchuk, *The Web That Has No Weaver* (New York: McGraw Hill, 2000), 437.

10. Kaptchuk, *The Web That Has No Weaver*, 438.

balance and optimize metabolic processes. In the following diagram of the Five Phases, the terms "generate" and "control" describe appropriate self-regulation between the functional systems, whereas the term "insult" describes a situation in which a functional system is overactive due to lack of control by another system. This creates abnormal symptoms in both areas of influence.

Diagram of the Five Phases

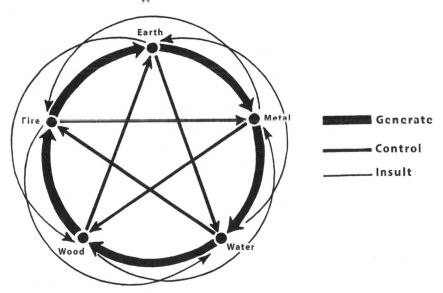

As long ago as the fourth century BCE, the Five Phases construct was used to understand and interrelate naturally occurring events. This understanding was applied to medicine as well as other disciplines, including astrology, politics, and the natural sciences.[11] Using this paradigm, Daoist physicians looked at the human body as a microcosm of the universe and sought to use the natural laws of the universe to maintain a harmonious balance. They believed that this balance must be maintained both within the patient and between the patient and the external environment. Following the principles of Daoism, which emphasize moderation and

---

11. Joseph Helms, *Acupuncture Energetics: A Clinical Approach for Physicians* (Berkeley, CA: Medical Acupuncture Publishers, 1995), 17.

equilibrium, the patient would be cautioned to follow the middle path in all aspects of life: to rest but also exercise, to work but have time for leisure, to eat a variety of healthy foods but neither too much nor too little. By achieving this equilibrium, the movement of the intelligent vital force within the body (called qi) would be smooth. This free movement of qi would maintain optimal health.

In 1973, in the Chinese province of Hunan, a famous archeological dig discovered silk texts that discussed subjects as diverse as astrology, art, military strategy, philosophy, and medicine. There were even two copies of Laozi's *Dao De Ching* found in the Mawangdui tombs (King Ma's Mound). Scientific methods were used to date the texts from approximately 200 BCE, and the tomb itself had been sealed in 168 BCE. The medical texts cover physiology, illness, surgery, herbal treatments, and what has been translated as "macrobiotic hygiene." Macrobiotic hygiene involves not only the body but also the spirit; this section discusses longevity, sexuality, and diet. Breathing and physical exercises are recommended for treating illness and cultivating health, and there are also writings on magic and incantations.[12]

Illness is described in the Mawangdui medical manuscripts as being the result of a disturbance in the movement of qi within the eleven vessels of the body. These vessels that contain qi are different from the arteries and veins that contain blood. The treatment advocated at the time involved cauterization of the qi vessels. There is no mention of using acupuncture needles to correct the flow of qi. Instead, the medical practitioners who wrote these manuscripts advocated the use of food, herbs, breath control, and exercise to improve the flow of qi and achieve a long and vibrant life.

This approach to good health was formalized in the classic medical text of the Han dynasty (206 BCE–220 CE), the *Huang Di Nei Jing* (*The Yellow Emperor's Classic of Internal Medicine*). It is thought that this text is a compilation of medical writings from practitioners of earlier centuries, which takes the form of a discussion between the Yellow Emperor (Huang Di) and his minister; it is significant in that it was the first known text to move away from shamanism and supernatural causes of disease. Like the Mawangdui medical manuscripts, the *Huang Di Nei Jing* discusses the

---

12. Donald J. Harper, *Early Chinese Medical Literature: The Mawangdui Medical Manuscripts* (London: Routledge, Taylor, and Francis, 1998), 6.

prevention and treatment of illness through diet, exercise, and herbs. Acupuncture theory is well described in the second volume of this text. The principles of energy flow within the body (qi), yin-yang theory, and diagnostic techniques are also discussed.

Around the first century BCE, the art of acupuncture using metal needles was formalized. Some researchers of Chinese medical history state that acupuncture arose from the practice of using sharpened stones and bones to lance infected skin, allowing the body to heal. However, scholars such as Paul Unschuld and Donald Harper state that the vessel theory and treatment paradigm delineated in the Mawangdui medical manuscripts was the necessary precursor to acupuncture theory as described in the *Huang Di Nei Jing*.[13]

Through trial and error, the Chinese determined that placing acupuncture needles at specific sites would give consistent and reproducible results. By the time the *Huang Di Nei Jing* was written, the intricate system of acupuncture points and qi flow within acupuncture channels was well established. Twelve paired principal channels, or vessels, were described, meaning that the channels were duplicated on each side of the body in a mirror image. These paired channels are named for organs of the body. The channels are Kidney, Heart, Small Intestine, Urinary Bladder, Spleen, Lung, Large Intestine, Stomach, Liver, *San Jiao*,[14] Pericardium,[15] and Gallbladder.

The channels can directly influence the named organ, but they also affect other areas and physiological processes. Additionally, eight "extraordinary" channels were noted. These special channels run in various directions, over and through the body, connecting the principal channels with reservoirs of qi known as the dan tian. The term dan tian translates into English as "elixir field."

There are three dan tian: the upper, middle, and lower. They are all located on the torso, but the upper dan tian also includes the head. The upper dan tian is located at the forehead. It is said to be the field in which the spirit resides. The middle dan tian is located at the solar plexus and is the storehouse of qi that is derived from the air you breathe and the food

---

13. Harper, *Early Chinese Medical Literature*, 5.
14. Also known as Triple Heater or Triple Burner.
15. Also known as Master of the Heart.

The Body Channels

Two Centerline Channels
Conception Vessel (Con)
Governing Vessel (Gov)

Twelve Principal Channels
Stomach Channel (Sto)
Spleen Channel (Spl)
Small Intestine Channel (SmI)
Heart Channel (Hea)
Bladder Channel (Bla)
Kidney Channel (Kid)
Pericardium Channel (Per)
Triple Warmer Channel (TrW)
Gall Bladder Channel (GaB)
Liver Channel (Liv)
Lung Channel (Lun)
Large Intestine Channel (LaI)

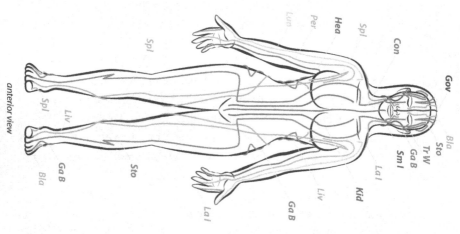

anterior view

Illustration courtesy of Shutterstock.

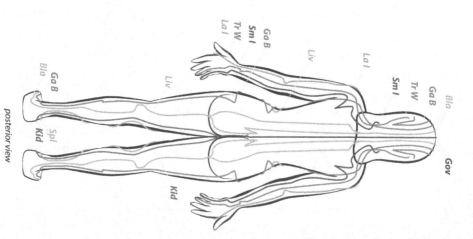

posterior view

you eat. This sort of qi is called "post-birth" or "post-heaven" qi because it is dependent upon your daily habits—sleep, diet, and exercise. The middle dan tian is also associated with feelings and emotions. The lower dan tian is located below the navel at the bottom of the torso. This dan tian is considered to be the "well spring" of human qi and is the reservoir of "pre-birth" or "pre-heaven"[16] qi. It is akin to your genetic constitution, the tendencies toward either health or disease that you received from your parents. The care that you take in cultivating your "post-birth qi" can enhance your overall health, even if your "pre-birth qi" carries a predisposition toward disease. In modern medicine, we have seen this born out in the study of epigenetics. Adequate sleep, nutrition, and exercise create conditions in the body for a change in genetic expression such that inherited tendencies toward diseases like diabetes, high blood pressure, and cancers may be avoided.

The three dan tian are connected by the extraordinary channels that act as conduits between the dan tian and the twelve principal channels. As seen in the previous diagram, there are two centerline channels called the conception vessel (also known as the ren mai) and governing vessel (the du mai). These are two of the eight extraordinary channels and connect the three dan tian. Another of the extraordinary channels is called the thrusting or penetrating vessel (chong mai). The penetrating vessel connects the lower dan tian to the upper dan tian through one of its five branches that ascends the spinal cord from the lower abdomen and pelvis to the brain. Another branch of the penetrating vessel communicates with the middle dan tian. The relationship between the dan tian, the extraordinary channels, and the principal channels and organs is very intricate. Acupuncture can influence the extraordinary channels and enhance the distribution of qi throughout the body. Acupuncture theory and science are discussed in more detail later in this chapter.

As in all ancient civilizations, the Chinese used indigenous plants, minerals, and animals as medicine. Chinese herbology predates acupuncture, probably by thousands of years, but until the development of written language, the use of these medicinals was not documented. Several very

---

16. Dr. Yang, Jwing-Ming, *The Root of Chinese Qigong* (Wolfeboro, NH: YMAA Publication Center, 1997), 33.

famous texts categorize Chinese herbs and explain their functions. *Shen Nong Ben Cao Jing* (*The Divine Farmer's Materia Medica*) was written in the early Tang dynasty (452–536 CE), but it is actually a compilation of much earlier writings. The book discusses the attributes of 365 herbs, the majority of which are still used today.

Dr. Zhang Zhong Jin (150–219 CE) was renowned for his text, the *Shang Han Lun* (*Treatise on Cold Damage*), the oldest formulary to group patient symptoms into clinically useful categories. Zhang Zhong Jin was also the first to link diagnoses derived through the principles of yin-yang theory and the Wu Xing (Five Phases) with standardized herbal treatments.

One of the most celebrated physicians in the history of Chinese medicine was Dr. Li Shi Zhen, who lived during the Ming dynasty. Li Shi Zhen traveled across China in search of medicinal herbs. In 1578, after twenty-seven years of diligent work, he completed his masterpiece, the *Ben Cao Gang Mu* (*Compendium of Materia Medica*). It documents 1,892 distinct herbs and more than eleven thousand formulas. This comprehensive text remained the official materia medica in China for the next four hundred years.

Two other noteworthy Chinese doctors are Hua Tuo (145–203 CE) and Sun Si-Miao (581–683 CE). Hua Tuo was well known, especially for his surgical skills and the development of a particular type of exercise that he called Five Animal Play (Wu Qin Xi). Sun Si-Miao stands out not only for his talent as a healer, but also for his humanity. Although the emperors of the Tang dynasty wanted Sun Si-Miao as the palace physician, he declined and worked for all people. In his writings, he instructed doctors to be of good moral character and to treat all patients equally, regardless of their class or wealth.

Around the time of Sun Si-Miao, during the fifth and sixth centuries, Eastern medicine spread from China to Japan, Korea, and Vietnam. Through trade via the Silk Road, knowledge of this system of medicine eventually arrived in the Middle East and Europe. As European colonization of East Asia increased, more Western physicians became curious about these techniques. For example, France had colonized Vietnam, and so French physicians who traveled there were exposed to the successes of acupuncture and herbal formulas. Other European countries followed suit. As early as 1700, there were references to acupuncture in the essays and books of physicians from France, Holland, Germany, Italy, and England.[17]

In the 1800s, American and Canadian physicians made note of acupuncture in their writings. In 1892, Dr. William Osler, a Canadian physician and one of the four founders of the Johns Hopkins Hospital, recommended the use of acupuncture for low back pain in his renowned text, *Principles and Practices of Medicine*.[18]

In the early twentieth century, the French diplomat, George Soulie de Morant, worked ceaselessly to promote the use of acupuncture. Soulie de Morant was not a doctor, though he had considered a career in medicine in his youth. While working in China, he saw acupuncture successfully used in treatment of cholera.[19] He was intrigued by acupuncture and Chinese medicine, and set about studying the craft. On his return to France, he eventually published *L'Acupuncture Chinoise* ("Chinese Acupuncture"). This text greatly influenced the practice of acupuncture in France and, later, in the United States. Soulie de Morant is considered the father of modern acupuncture and his writings and lectures set the stage for research into the mechanisms of action of this modality. In fact, the French were at the forefront of Western investigations of Eastern medicine. Later in this chapter, we discuss the science of acupuncture and other Eastern healing modalities in greater detail.

An increasing percentage of the world population has benefited from Eastern medicine over the past century, but in the United States very few were able to take advantage of this powerful medical system prior to the 1970s. Until then, acupuncture was illegal in America. Even though it was utilized and well respected throughout Japan and other Asian countries, Europe, Britain, and Canada, both practitioners and patients who sought to use this medicine risked arrest in the United States. For this reason, very little documentation remains of the early history of Eastern medicine in America. There are, however, some accounts dating as far back as the nineteenth century. In 1974, California became the first state to legalize the practice of acupuncture, after which most other states began to follow suit. Acupuncture training and credentialing became more formalized,

---

17. Birch and Felt, *Understanding Acupuncture*, 45.
18. Birch and Felt, 49.
19. Birch and Felt, 191.

but there are still a few states in which there is no regulation of acupuncture practice. In all states except Hawai'i, a medical doctor or osteopath may practice acupuncture after completing approximately three hundred hours of acupuncture training; such a practitioner is called a medical acupuncturist. A licensed acupuncturist is not usually a medical doctor or osteopath, although some physicians choose to enroll in schools of acupuncture and Eastern medicine. Licensed acupuncturists usually have some post-secondary education and then will have completed approximately three thousand hours of training in acupuncture and herbology. This also would include hundreds of hours of courses in Western biomedicine such as anatomy, biology, chemistry, physiology, and pharmacology.

Whether a medical or licensed acupuncturist, the mark of an excellent practitioner is their willingness to refine the art and science of Eastern medicine. Collaboration among acupuncturists and other healthcare practitioners is happening more frequently in clinics, hospitals, and academic institutions. The drive to comprehend the mechanism of action of acupuncture, qigong, taiji, yoga, and meditation has fueled thousands of basic research studies and clinical trials. In the discussion that follows, we provide a brief summary of the current understanding of how these therapies can heal the human body.

The Science behind Eastern Healing Modalities

From Asia to Europe to the rest of the world, interest in and use of Eastern medicine has grown during the past century, surging over the last fifty years. Several components of Eastern medicine have been subject to scientific scrutiny not only in the West, but also in their countries of origin. The elements of Eastern medicine (including Indian, Tibetan, and Chinese practices) that have been most researched are meditation and breath control, yoga, qigong, taiji, herbal remedies, and acupuncture.

Regulation of the breath has been used for millennia to calm the mind and heal the body. Even without a modern understanding of how the brain and body communicate, the ancients formulated breathing techniques that balanced the autonomic nervous system. The autonomic nervous system controls activities you don't have to think about. These activities are called involuntary. For example, you don't need to think about breathing in and out, keeping your heart beating, or digesting your food. To keep everything running smoothly, your autonomic system can adjust all these bodily functions through the interaction of your brain, peripheral nerves, immune system, and endocrine system. The autonomic nervous system is composed of the sympathetic nervous system and the parasympathetic nervous system. The sympathetic nervous system initiates the release of stress hormones when your brain perceives that you are in danger. These hormones cause your heart rate to elevate, your blood pressure to rise, and makes glucose available to fuel your muscles in preparation for combat or evasive maneuvers. This reaction is known as the fight-or-flight response. In contrast, the parasympathetic nervous system calms all these processes and returns the body to a normal state of activity. Slow, deep breathing stimulates the main nerve of the parasympathetic nervous system, called the vagus nerve, which in turn releases hormones and neurotransmitters that slow your heart rate, lower your blood pressure, and generally bring your body into balance.[20] The benefits of calming the nervous system include decreasing chronic inflammation, thereby decreasing your risk of chronic illness.

Controlling the breath is often one of the first steps employed in meditation. There are many different types of meditation—Buddhist, Hindu, Zen, Tibetan, Daoist, mindfulness, and many more. Depending on the ideology associated with the practice, the goals of meditation can range from relaxation and stress relief to compassion and spiritual enlightenment. Meditation usually results in a sense of calmness and clarity that can be difficult to describe. Numerous medical benefits have been attributed to meditation, and scientists are investigating how meditation affects the brain and overall health.

---

20. T. M. Srinivasan, "Pranayama and Brain Correlates," *Ancient Science of Life* 11, no. 1/2 (1991): 1–6; D. Krshnakumar, M. R. Hamblin, and S. Lakshmanan, "Meditation and Yoga Can Modulate Brain Mechanisms That Affect Behaviour and Anxiety," *Ancient Science of Life* 2, no.1 (2015): 13–19, https://doi.org/10.14259/as/ v2i2il1.171; Michael M. Zanoni, "Healing Resonance Qi Gong and Hamanaleo Meditation," https://www.mikezanoni.com/meditation-qi-gong, accessed February 4, 2018.

When a person meditates, the electrical activity in the brain changes. This is true of any change of state such as intense concentration or emotion, drowsiness, sleep, and dreaming. These patterns of electrical activity are called brain waves and are measured by electroencephalography (EEG). Brain waves, also known as neural oscillations, have different frequencies. In addition, a wide range of patterns, combinations of frequencies, and amplitudes are associated with different stages of sleep and wakefulness. For instance, you can be awake and in a state of deep concentration as you are trying to solve a problem or you can be awake but daydreaming and inattentive. Each of these states of wakefulness has different patterns involving each of the frequencies but in different proportions and can involve different areas of the brain. Simply stated, higher-frequency brain waves are associated with cognitive processing and alertness (beta waves); lower frequencies are associated with sleep (delta waves). In between, there are frequencies associated with wakefulness (alpha waves) and deep relaxation, daydreaming, and meditation (theta waves). Combinations of delta and theta waves are important in memory processing. The state of mind between alpha and theta waves is said to be one of increased creativity.

Through the use of functional magnetic resonance imaging (fMRI), researchers have discovered that meditation increases the amount of gray matter in the brain, which is made up predominantly of the cell bodies of the neurons,[21] and also seems to slow the natural loss of gray matter that occurs as we age.[22] Depending on the location of the gray matter within the brain, it is involved with a variety of functions such as learning, memory, emotional regulation, and perspective. It seems that meditation can actually keep your brain younger and calmer.

A meditative state can be achieved during qigong, taiji, and yoga. All these practices incorporate slow deep-breathing patterns, which confer all the benefits of seated meditation. These forms of moving meditation have additional advantages. During these practices, we move in well-defined

---

21. Britta K. Holzel et al., "Mindfulness Practice Leads to Increases in Regional Brain Gray Matter Density," *Psychiatry Research* 191, no.1 (2011): 36–43, https//doi.org/10:1016/j.pscychresns.2010.08.006.

22. N. Last, E. Tufts, and L. E. Auger, "The Effects of Meditation on Grey Matter Atrophy and Neurodegeneration: A Systematic Review," *Journal of Alzheimer's Disease* 56, no.1 (2017): 275–286, https://doi.org/10.3233/JAD-160899.

patterns, stretching all the muscles in the neck, torso, arms, and legs. Stretching has many benefits, such as decreasing pain, improving blood circulation, increasing range of motion, and improving balance. For some time now, the cellular changes that occur with stretching have been studied. Dr. Helene Langevin, who in 2018 was appointed as the director of the National Center for the Complementary and Integrative Health (NCCIH), demonstrated that by gently stretching the connective tissue of mice, inflammation at a site of injury was reduced. There was also an increase in the concentration of resolvins, the cellular mediators that help coordinate the resolution of the acute inflammatory episode.[23] In another study, using a similar rodent model and injecting breast cancer cells into the mice, Dr. Langevin found that gentle connective tissue stretching enhanced the response of the immune system and slowed the tumor growth by half.[24] This finding may offer an explanation for why many researchers have noted a lower risk of death from all causes, including recurrence, in cancer patients who exercise.[25]

An additional benefit of slow-moving, breath-focused exercise relates to the way the body utilizes oxygen. Dr. Peter Anthony Gryffin has compared the amount of oxygen in the blood during and after aerobic exercises such as running and after slow, mindful exercises like taiji and qigong. It was previously known that the amount of oxygen in the blood, a measurement called blood oxygen saturation, either stays the same or goes down during aerobic exercise as oxygen is being utilized by the large muscle groups, heart, and lungs. During slow-moving, breath-focused exercises, blood oxygen saturation initially goes up, then drops significantly for a short period of time before returning to baseline. Dr. Gryffin's research suggests that this drop in blood oxygen saturation represents

---

23. L. Berrueta et al., "Stretching Impacts Inflammation Resolution in Connective Tissue," *Journal of Cellular Physiology* 231, no. 7 (2016): 1621–1627, https://doi.org/10.1002/jcp.25623.

24. L. Berrueta et al., "Stretching Reduces Tumor Growth in a Mouse Breast Cancer Model," *Scientific Reports* 8, 7864 (2018), https://doi.org/10.1038/s41598-018-26198-7.

25. David O. Garcia and Cynthia A. Thomson, "Physical Activity and Cancer Survivorship," *Nutrition in Clinical Practice* 29, no. 6 (2014): 768–779, https://doi.org/10.1177/0884533614551969.

increased oxygen metabolism and diffusion throughout the whole body, since no excessive strain is placed on the muscles and cardiovascular system, as occurs during aerobic exercise. Because of this unique difference in oxygen metabolism, Dr. Gryffin coined the term "metarobics" to describe exercises that are neither aerobic, like running or swimming, nor anaerobic, like weightlifting. Metarobic exercises include taiji, qigong, yoga, and other forms of moving meditation. This improved oxygen metabolism may account for many of the health benefits realized by practitioners of taiji and qigong, such as decreased levels of chronic inflammation, improved immunity, and enhanced healing.[26]

Along with meditation, breath regulation, and movement, herbs are a mainstay in Eastern medicine, as well as in every medical tradition around the world. The healing properties of plants have been known for thousands of years, but not until the last two hundred years have specific biologically active compounds been extracted and used as drugs. As technology advanced, the medicinal properties of herbs were documented, particularly in China, where sophisticated combinations of herbs are used alongside modern pharmaceuticals in clinics and hospitals that integrate Western and Eastern care modalities. The constituent components of these herbs, the ways they are metabolized, and how they affect the body continue to be documented. These plants have naturally occurring compounds that, depending on the herb, can act as antibacterials, antivirals, antifungals, hormone modulators, neurotransmitters, anti-inflammatories, antidepressants, or sleep aids. It is not within the scope of this book to discuss the biochemistry of all the herbs available to a qualified practitioner, but it should be noted that many of the formulas around today have been prescribed effectively in Asia for more than a thousand years.

The concept of using plants as medicines was well established throughout the world, but it was the mystery of acupuncture that fascinated the French. When Soulie de Morant started to introduce acupuncture to Western physicians, one of the difficulties he encountered was the translation of concepts from Chinese to French and other languages. Soulie de

---

26. Peter Anthony Gryffin, *Mindful Exercise: Metarobics, Healing, and the Power of Tai Chi* (Wolfeboro, NH: YMAA Publication Center, 2018), 15.

Morant was fluent in Chinese, having studied it since he was a child. Moreover, he lived in China for decades and understood the cultural nuances. When it came to translating the word "qi," Soulie de Morant chose to liken it to a popular concept at the time, the *elan vital* (human energy).[27] He felt that Western physicians would more easily accept the concept that energy within the body was modulated by acupuncture since early twentieth century medicine had already discovered nerve impulses. This led to various scientific experiments that attempted to discover the mechanism of action of acupuncture and further define and quantify qi, which helped to lay the foundation for modern acupuncture research.

As we embark on an overview of acupuncture research over the past century, it will help to conceptualize qi not only as energy, but also as an information signaling system that exists within the matrix of the human body. In their book, *Understanding Acupuncture*, Stephen Birch and Robert Felt describe qi as "a model of universal order and communication,"[28] where qi is at once the matrix of information and the process of its exchange.[29] As we shall see, there is no single, simple explanation for acupuncture's mechanism of action or method to quantify qi. Each scientist, and there have been many, added new information, helping to fill in the pieces of the puzzle.

In the 1940s and 1950s, Dr. J. E. H. Niboyet designed a series of experiments that showed electrical resistance is lower at acupuncture points than elsewhere on the body. This means electricity will pass into the body more easily across the skin at an acupuncture point than across the skin at a non-acupuncture point. Niboyet also demonstrated that electricity flowed more easily along the same acupuncture channel than between channels that were not as strongly related to each other. These results were confirmed by other scientists in the 1960s and 1970s, but subsequent studies by Andrew Ahn in the early twenty-first century demonstrate that

---

27. Birch and Felt, *Understanding Acupuncture*, 105.
28. Birch and Felt, 109.
29. Rosa N. Schnyer, DAOM, personal communication with author (CK), Dec. 17, 2019.

decreased electrical resistance is more consistently found along acupuncture channels than the points themselves.[30][31]

The acupuncture channel itself has remained an elusive entity. Our understanding of acupuncture channels and how acupuncture works has changed over time. Acupuncture channels are intimately associated with the neural, immune, and endocrine systems of the body. Understanding that some of the effects of acupuncture are mediated via electricity was the first step in uncovering its mechanism of action. Over the past half century, the uncovering of this knowledge began by seeking evidence that these channels do exist: they were thought to be different than the known vascular or neurological systems that have been defined by modern medicine. The first piece of indirect evidence of the existence of acupuncture channels is that many patients experience a feeling of heaviness, achiness, or warmth around the acupuncture needles during treatments. These sensations can radiate from the needles, either circumferentially or linearly. When moving linearly, this feeling of warmth or achiness travels up or down the area of the body being needled. Modern Chinese researchers call this phenomenon "propagated sensation along channels."[32] They suggest that the sensation represents the movement of a corrective signal to an area determined by the acupuncture point. The target zone for the propagated sensation need not be a local area. Needling particular points on an arm or leg can reproducibly create a response in another part of the body. For example, certain points on the hand can alleviate back pain, a point on the lower leg can decrease discomfort of the opposite shoulder, and a well-known combination of points can initiate labor. We do know that the sensations elicited by acupuncture are an essential part of the signaling process and are caused by the activation of different types of nerve fibers.[33]

The speed of the propagated sensation travels at one to ten centimeters per second. This velocity varies among subjects and with the intensity of

---

30. Joseph Helms, *Acupuncture Energetics: A Clinical Approach for Physicians* (Berkeley, CA: Medical Acupuncture Publishers, 1995), 21.

31. Andrew C. Ahn et al, "Electrical Properties of Acupuncture Points and Meridians: A Systematic Review," *Bioelectromagnetics* 29 (2008): 245-256.

32. Helms, *Acupuncture Energetics*, 22.

33. Michael Corradino, *Neuropuncture: A Clinical Handbook of Neuroscience Acupuncture*, 2nd ed. (London: Singing Dragon, 2013), 24.

the needling. The rate is much, much slower than the speed of nerve impulses, so it cannot be attributed simply to nerve conduction. The brain itself is also involved in the perception of this sensation. Some studies have reported that amputees who are aware of phantom limbs are able to feel the propagated sensation within the absent limb when needled along a channel associated with the limb in question. This indicates that there must be some central nervous system involvement in the appreciation of this sensation.

When an acupuncture point is needled, a lot happens on the cellular level. There seem to be other mechanisms at play, aside from direct activation of the nervous system. When the needle is inserted, it is manipulated to create sensation. This manipulation causes a mechanical change in the tissue. Researchers have demonstrated, using magnetic resonance imaging and ultrasound elastography, that a slow-moving wave is generated through the tissue that has been needled. There is also a shift in calcium ions that creates a biochemical signal that appears to be separate from the electrical signal of the nerve fibers.[34]

Western science has added a great deal of supporting evidence for the existence of a communication network from acupuncture points to the rest of the body by documenting the effects of acupuncture on blood chemistry, body temperature, and hormone levels. With respect to blood chemistry, acupuncture has been shown to modify levels of glucose, cortisol, triglycerides, and cholesterol. Although the mechanism of action is not well understood, acupuncture seems to assist the body in achieving balance. In medicine, this equilibrium is called homeostasis.

Acupuncture has also been shown to increase the body's surface temperature by causing the blood vessels to dilate, resulting in increased blood flow. The increase has been documented at a rate three times higher than that of pretreatment flow. Not only does the surface temperature of the needled skin increase locally, but it also increases at the same area on the other side of the body.[35] Increased blood flow improves oxygenation within the tissue and may speed healing.

---

34. Edward S. Yang et al., "Ancient Chinese Medicine and Mechanistic Evidence of Acupuncture Physiology," *European Journal of Physiology* 462 (2011): 645–653, https://doi.org/10.1007/s00424-011-1017-3.

35. Joseph Helms, *Acupuncture Energetics: A Clinical Approach for Physicians* (Berkeley, CA: Medical Acupuncture Publishers, 1995), 40.

There has been a great deal of research on acupuncture's effect on hormone and neurotransmitter levels, particularly with respect to pain relief. Some of these neurotransmitters include serotonin, norepinephrine, substance P, GABA (gamma-aminobutyric acid), and dopamine. All of these compounds work together to diminish the brain's perception of pain.

Another way that pain is decreased is through the release of cortisol, which has an anti-inflammatory action. The release of cortisol is controlled by levels of adrenocorticotrophic hormone (ACTH), and acupuncture has been shown to increase the discharge of this substance.

Finally, acupuncture modulates the body's internal production of opioids, leading to pain relief through a different pathway. Opioids are narcotic-like compounds; those produced in the body are called endorphins, which attach to receptors located on cell membranes, resulting in decreased pain. There are several different types of endorphins, and each acts at a different site within the brain and spinal cord to relieve pain. Interestingly, it appears that certain endorphins (beta-endorphin and met-enkephalin) also interact with the immune system. A surge in the levels of these endorphins can lead to increased activity of natural killer cells, a type of white blood cell that defends the body from foreign microbes and cancerous mutations.[36]

For all the various effects that acupuncture produces, the specific mechanism of action has not yet been completely discovered. As we have seen, electricity is a principal mediator of information that is passed along through the body, creating numerous physiologic changes.

There are several theories about how these processes are regulated. Most of them concentrate on the effects produced by the passage of electrical current through the body. There is no doubt the human body utilizes electricity in its everyday functioning. Western medicine has used this information to create many diagnostic tests and therapies.

In the heart, the interpretation of the electrical signals seen on an electrocardiogram (EKG) allows a physician to diagnose a heart attack or cardiac rhythm disturbance. If a patient's heart suddenly stops beating, electricity is applied to the person's chest via a device called a defibrillator

---

36. Helms, *Acupuncture Energetics*, 41.

in an effort to "kick-start" cardiac activity. Smaller amounts of electricity are also used to change irregular rhythms to regular ones.

The electrical signals from the brain can be studied to help diagnose epilepsy or sleep disturbances. We can assess the health of these systems by recording the speed of electrical impulses through the nerves and muscles.

Even skin healing, which we tend to take for granted, requires electricity to activate the restorative process. Electrically, the skin can be described as a battery, with the negative charge inside each cell and the positive charge on the exterior surface. When the skin is breached, either by trauma or by inserting an acupuncture needle, the "battery" is short-circuited, and the charge on the skin surface becomes negative. This negative charge seems to be an initiating factor in healing and activates the body's system of repair. It has been shown that this negative charge, described by Dr. Robert Becker as a "current of injury," can last several days following an acupuncture treatment.[37]

Dr. Becker, an American orthopedic surgeon, performed a fascinating series of experiments involving electrical current and limb regeneration in salamanders and frogs. Even though salamanders and frogs are closely related, salamanders can spontaneously regrow lost limbs, but frogs cannot. Through his research, Dr. Becker discovered that the tissue over the salamanders' limb stumps display a relatively negative charge compared with other points on the animal. The frogs did not exhibit this negative charge. When he applied the appropriate electrical current and created a negative charge over the area of the frogs' missing limbs, the frogs' limbs regenerated just like the salamanders' did.[38] Dr. Becker's work has led to the creation of electrical devices that accelerate bone healing. These devices are used in cases in which broken bones are not healing well. In the past, it was sometimes necessary to amputate limbs that would not heal. By using electricity to enhance bone healing, Dr. Becker's discovery has decreased the need for amputation in such circumstances.

In addition to the electrical component of the energy within the human body, there is also a magnetic component. Without this, magnetic resonance imaging (MRI) would not be possible. Studies called functional

---

37. Helms, 67.

38. Richard Gerber, *Vibrational Medicine: The #1 Handbook of Subtle-Energy Therapies*, 3rd ed. (Rochester, VT: Bear and Company, 2001), 91.

MRIs are used to observe the electromagnetic changes within different areas of the brain in response to acupuncture needling.

Other devices have been developed that can measure electromagnetic fields that come from diverse parts of the body. Such devices have demonstrated that electromagnetic fields exist around acupuncture points and that the intensity of these fields changes following acupuncture treatment.[39] Some researchers suggest that acupuncture points act as amplifiers by increasing the signal that moves along the channel.

Identifying the exact tissues through which these electromagnetic signals pass is a subject of ongoing study. Evidence suggests a variety of mechanisms through which bioelectrical information is transmitted. These mechanisms include:

- Electron-rich fluid that naturally bathes the tissues of the body, organized into tiny pockets now recognized as the interstitium, a newly defined organ[40]
- Perineural cells (cells that are adjacent to nerves)
- Proteins such as hormones and neurotransmitters that regulate communication between cells
- The fascia, a fibrous tissue that surrounds and connects every component of the body, from nerves, arteries, and veins to each muscle and organ

In his superb book *The Spark in the Machine*, Dr. Daniel Keown explains the role that fascia plays in the body, including its electrical properties. Fascia is composed of collagen. Collagen is a protein that accounts for 30 percent of the proteins in our body. Proteins are made of amino acids. In collagen fibers, these amino acids are arranged into three threads that twist around each other like three-stranded rope, lending incredible tensile strength to the tissues in which it is found; these include bones, ligaments, tendons, cartilage, arteries, and connective tissue. Just as it sounds,

---

39. Joseph Helms, *Acupuncture Energetics: A Clinical Approach for Physicians* (Berkeley, CA: Medical Acupuncture Publishers, 1995), 62.

40. Petros C. Benias et al., "Structure and Distribution of an Unrecognized Interstitium in Human Tissues," *Scientific Reports* 8, article no. 4947 (2018), https://doi.org/10.1038/s41598-018-23062-6.

connective tissue connects and surrounds all our organs and muscles. Collagen even creates the lattice of the interstitium and interacts directly with the fluid inside these bundles, potentially allowing communication between body systems.[41]

Dr. Keown explains that, because of its molecular structure, collagen can act like a crystal and generate small currents of piezoelectricity when it undergoes mechanical stress. If a substance is piezoelectric, it will generate a change in electrical charge when it is compressed and then returns to its original shape. We take advantage of piezoelectricity when we use pilot lights on a gas grill to create a spark, igniting the flame. Collagen is also a semiconductor. This means that collagen can conduct electricity, but not as well as metal such as copper. It can also act as an insulator, but not as well as glass. So, with every movement you make, your tendons, muscles, and bones undergo mechanical strain, and the collagen generates an electrical current. Collagen is an integral part of the fascia that connects the top of your head to the tip of your toes. Dr. Keown describes this as "an interconnected, living electrical web."[42]

When an acupuncture needle is inserted into the body, it makes contact with this "living electrical web." The acupuncturist will usually manipulate the needle until both the patient and the practitioner are aware of a certain sensation. The patient may feel an ache or a slight electrical zing at the insertion site, and this feeling may propagate along the body part that is needled. The acupuncturist can feel this through the needle. This sensation is called "de qi," or "the arrival of the qi." Even if the needle is inserted into an area that is not classified as an acupuncture point or is not along the channel, this sensation may be felt. This is because the fascia wraps the whole body, not only along acupuncture channels. Just as the blood flows through large vessels and tiny capillaries, so too does piezoelectricity traverse the whole body.

Knowing about the "body electric," researchers have tried to explain the location of acupuncture channels and points, forming hypotheses regarding the way in which bioelectromagnetic information travels through the body.

---

41. Benias et al., "Structure and Distribution of an Unrecognized Interstitium."
42. Daniel Keown, *The Spark in the Machine* (London: Singing Dragon, 2014), 21.

Chang-Lin Zhang and Fritz-Albert Popp theorize that electromagnetic energy travels in waves.[43] These waves bounce off the physical structures in the body such as bones, nerves, and skin, creating interference patterns, similar to the way waves of water reflect off the sides of a pool. As they change direction, the waves combine with others, creating higher waves, or canceling each other out. Zhang and Popp suggest that acupuncture points and channels occur at areas where bioelectromagnetic waves have combined to form new waves of higher amplitudes, and that acupuncture needles can be used to change the body's electromagnetic field.

Acupuncture needles may influence the state of the body through more than one single path. The human body is a complex system, and it seems likely that the ways in which acupuncture affects it are manifold. In an effort to tease apart the specific mechanism of action, researchers over the years have designed studies comparing true acupuncture with different sorts of pretend acupuncture, called sham acupuncture.

Sham acupuncture has been variously described as needling prescribed points superficially, needling non-acupuncture points, needling points that have not traditionally been used for the condition being treated, or using retractable needles to simulate the experience of true acupuncture without the actual needle insertion.

In numerous studies, sham acupuncture has been shown to be almost as effective as true acupuncture. Those that doubt the usefulness of acupuncture interpret this as placebo effect; however, when using shallow needling, alternate points, or retractable needles, the collagen in the connective tissue of the body is still compressed. The piezoelectric property of collagen is activated whenever these tissues are compressed, and microcurrents of electricity are generated. The body's response to the energetic input of sham acupuncture may not be as pronounced as when the points are actually needled, but the body responds nonetheless. This explains why, in some studies, sham acupuncture can be better than no treatment and almost as effective as "real" acupuncture, particularly if the sham acupuncture involves skin penetration. One interesting finding in a recent systematic review of acupuncture trials in the treatment of several types of chronic pain is that penetrating sham acupuncture more closely

---

43. Helms, *Acupuncture Energetics*, 69.

approximates the pain-relieving effect of true acupuncture than does the non-penetrating sham.[44]

Prior to our clearer understanding of the physiological effects of acupuncture, many considered the improvements patients experienced to be the result of a placebo effect, which has been seen in medical practice for centuries. The word "placebo" comes from the Latin meaning "to please." The idea was that a doctor would give a patient a pill or treatment that was inert. If a pill, there was no active substance in it; if a treatment or surgery, there was no actual intentional repair of any structure. In spite of this, a large number of patients actually improved or were cured. Placebos were historically used to encourage the patient's expectation that they would recover. Researchers use placebos to ensure that the experience that both the study group and the control group undergo is as close to the same as possible. The goal is to isolate the one active substance or intervention that is creating a change in the patient's condition. Introducing a placebo group into a randomized controlled trial is common, but as we have seen, sometimes placebos confuse rather than clarify the results.

Even when a study involves a simple cause-and-effect response, such as testing a new drug, it is impossible to separate the human reactions of the participants, both patients and researchers. Medical anthropologists like Cecil Helman have pointed out for some time that there is a "total effect" of a drug or intervention that goes beyond the actual biochemical or physiologic nature of the treatment. The components that make up the total effect include the characteristics of the drug or treatment itself (even down to the color of the pill), the characteristics of the patient (age, gender, genetics, education, experience, personality, expectations), the characteristics of the researcher (personality, age, gender, attitude, professional status), and the setting in which the study is taking place.[45]

None of the above attributes can be removed from the clinical trial, and all of these characteristics are present within the study and placebo

---

44. A. J. Vickers et al., "Acupuncture for Chronic Pain: Update of an Individual Patient Data Meta-Analysis," *Journal of Pain* 19, no. 5 (2018): 455–474, https://doi.org/10.1016/j.jpain.2017.11.005.

45. Elisabeth Hsu, "Treatment Evaluation: An Anthropologist's Approach," in *Integrating East Asian Medicine into Contemporary Health Care*, ed. Volker Scheid and Hugh MacPherson (Edinburgh: Churchill Livingstone/Elsevier, 2012), 158.

groups. This may, in part, explain why some patients who receive the active substance experience a negative clinical response and some within the placebo group improve.

So, does this mean that the positive clinical results experienced by placebo group patients are a figment of their imagination? No. In many studies, the improvements seen in the placebo group can be objectively identified. These changes are not just qualitative, meaning the patient describes a state of improved health. The differences can also be defined quantitatively, such as findings of lower blood pressure and lower cholesterol levels, and the decreased use of painkillers.

How can these changes be occurring? There is a great deal of interest in physiologic effects of the placebo. Around the world, researchers are documenting changes that occur in the immune system, the brain, the spinal cord, and the biochemical balance of the body in response to a placebo.

In many of these studies, patients are not told they are receiving a placebo. For many, this presents an ethical dilemma in the use of placebos in general practice. Interestingly, at Harvard's Program for Placebo Studies, Kaptchuk and others created a randomized controlled trial to look at the feasibility of using placebos without deceiving the patient.[46] All the patients had irritable bowel syndrome (IBS). The patients were randomized either to the open-label placebo group or the nontreatment control. Both groups received the same amount of time, counseling, and attention. Both groups were asked not to change any aspect of their usual routines for the duration of the study, such as starting a new diet or exercise program. Both groups had stable disease. The difference came at the end of the first interview, when the patients found out to which group they were assigned. The open-label group was told the pills they would take were "placebos, made of an inert substance, like sugar pills, that have been shown in clinical studies to produce significant improvement in IBS symptoms through mind-body self-healing processes."

The truly fascinating outcome of Kaptchuk's study was that, even though patients knew they were taking placebos, their IBS symptoms improved more than those of the control group, which did not receive any

---

46. T. J. Kaptchuk et al., "Placebos without Deception: A Randomized Controlled Trial in Irritable Bowel Syndrome," *PLoS* One 5, no. 12 (2010): e15591, doi:10.1371/journal.pone.0015591.

pills. The statistically significant changes in the study group were decreased symptom severity and increased symptom relief. There was also a trend toward improved quality-of-life scores at the end of the study period for those taking placebos. Remember that these patients knew there was no medication of any sort in their pills, and yet they felt better. This demonstrates that the power of the mind to heal the body is astonishing. Eastern medicine has always recognized that fact and uses it to full advantage by incorporating meditation, qigong, and taiji into patient care. Further research will shed more light on this intriguing phenomenon. Even though the mechanism of action is not fully understood, we can still benefit from the positive physiologic changes that acupuncture and mind-body interventions produce.

Western Health-Care Providers and Eastern Medicine

Conventionally trained physicians all over the world are seeking ways to help their patients move toward optimal health. There is a strong sense among Western healthcare providers that pharmaceutical and surgical interventions may not be enough to correct the course of modern diseases, the majority of which are caused by poor lifestyle choices. There is no doubt that under certain circumstances, medications and surgery can be lifesaving; however, medicine often does not get to the root of the problem and only acts as a temporary fix. Increasingly, doctors, physician assistants, and nurse practitioners recommend integrating complementary therapies into regular medical care.

Even without the input of a healthcare provider, people are choosing to use supplements, herbs, and treatments that are not considered standard in Western medicine. The National Institutes of Health (NIH) regularly conducts surveys of tens of thousands of adults regarding their use of complementary or alternative medicine; approximately one-third of those surveyed use these therapies. Western practitioners now commonly ask their patients if they are using any other supplements, herbs, or alternative healing modalities. In fact, medical students are now taught to ask these questions as a matter of course, and academic health centers for integrative medicine can be found in such prestigious schools as Harvard, Tufts, Stanford, the University of Toronto, and the Mayo Clinic, to name but a few. Medical students are now learning about other traditional health systems so they can understand how these treatments can be safely integrated into conventional care. Hospitals are also offering complementary and integrative healing services. The American Hospital Association released a survey in 2011 demonstrating that 42 percent of their member hospitals provided these modalities, representing an increase from 37 percent in 2007.[47]

These complementary therapies cover a wide range of options and healing systems. Depending on practitioners' interests and experience, they may suggest adjunctive Western therapies such as biofeedback, relaxation techniques, massage therapy, health coaching, and lifestyle medicine programs. Or they might consider Ayurvedic medicine that incorporates yoga, meditation, herbs, and dietary therapies based on the patient's underlying constitution. Yet again, they may refer their patients to a practitioner of Eastern medicine. Like other healing systems, Eastern medicine is composed of various strands: dietary therapy, exercise, qigong, taiji, meditation, bodywork, herbal formulas, and acupuncture. All of these complementary therapies are aimed at improving the physical, mental, and emotional health of the patient and modifying underlying behaviors that contribute to chronic disease.

Many medical practitioners and patients will have preferences regarding which therapeutic interventions to use. After discussing the options, they may decide to stick with one traditional system entirely or mix and match depending on circumstances. For example, someone may respond well to Ayurvedic dietary therapy but have mobility problems and find it too difficult to get down on the floor to practice yoga. That person might do better with taiji or qigong. Both of these Eastern practices will improve strength and balance as well as provide the preparation for meditation that yoga confers.

---

47. American Hospital Association, "More Hospitals Offering Complementary and Alternative Medicine Services," September 7, 2011, https://www.aha.org/press-releases/2011-09-07-more-hospitals-offering-complementary-and-alternative-medicine-services.

We too have our preferences. Our training in both Western and Eastern medicine has shown us that these two systems work extremely well together, and we are not alone. Over the span of two decades, the percentage of Western physicians who had a favorable opinion of Eastern medicine increased fourfold. In 1998, only 20 percent of respondents held a positive view of Eastern medicine. When the survey was repeated in 2009, that number had exploded to 80 percent![48]

Even the United States military has embraced a component of Eastern medicine. In 2007, the US Air Force asked Dr. Joseph Helms, the founding president of the American Academy of Medical Acupuncture, to develop acupuncture protocols to treat conditions commonly found in combat veterans: post-traumatic stress disorder (PTSD) and pain, both acute and chronic. From 2008 to 2013, the US Department of Defense funded medical acupuncture training for hundreds of military doctors under the guidance of Dr. Helms. When this funding was no longer available, Dr. Helms created the Acus Foundation, a not-for-profit charitable organization, to continue training military healthcare providers in medical acupuncture. Acus partnered with Nellis Air Force Base, training all the primary-care physicians so that any patient could receive an acupuncture treatment at any visit upon request or recommendation. In the first year of this pilot program, opioid prescriptions dropped by 45 percent, muscle relaxant prescriptions decreased by 34 percent, and $250,000 was saved thanks to fewer referrals to civilian pain-management specialists.[49]

Although you may not have access to a primary-care provider who is also a skilled acupuncturist, you can rest assured that a great many Western physicians are genuinely interested in incorporating Eastern therapies into conventional medical care. Your doctor may already know a number of reputable practitioners of Eastern medicine and would be happy to refer you. Some patients are reluctant to bring up the topic of incorporating Eastern medicine into their usual treatment plan. They are worried that

---

48. From the keynote address of the 2011 American Academy of Medical Acupuncture Symposium, given by Emmeline Edwards, MD, director of the Division of Extramural Research at the National Center for Complementary and Integrative Health, a component of the NIH, March 2011.

49. Acus Foundation, https://acusfoundation.org/our-programs/teaching/, accessed June 13, 2018.

they will offend their doctors. In this day and age, with all the emerging evidence demonstrating the effectiveness of acupuncture, meditative practices, and lifestyle changes, most physicians are open to adding these strategies to regular care. If your doctor *is* offended, we respectfully suggest you find a new primary care provider.

You will not know how your doctor feels about integrating Eastern and Western medicine until you have the conversation. As we discussed in our first book, *True Wellness*, there may be several reasons that your primary care provider has not spoken to you about these modalities. It may be that your doctor doesn't know whether Eastern medicine would be useful for your particular condition. Or she may not have access to reliable practitioners of Eastern medicine to whom she can send you. Or she may not want to suggest a therapy that might incur additional costs to you if your health insurance doesn't cover these services. These reasons should not prevent you from discussing treatment options with your doctor.

To have a meaningful discussion, you should come to the appointment prepared. You need to do a little homework. Since the inception of the internet, most physicians are very comfortable with patients who have done some online research about their illness and are happy to go through the downloaded information with you. If you are going to present your doctor with such information, it is important that it has come from reputable sources. The World Health Organization report on acupuncture is a good place to start. You could also search the websites of several prominent medical centers that offer Eastern medical services and see what conditions they commonly treat.

You should call your health insurance company to see whether Eastern medical services are a covered benefit and, if so, which providers are in the network. If this option is unavailable to you, you can cover the expense yourself, understanding that within three to five treatments you will know whether they are beneficial. If you live near a school of Eastern medicine, there will be a community clinic where you can receive care for a reduced cost.

Now that you have determined for yourself whether Eastern medicine is a suitable modality for your condition and how to access that care, you will feel more comfortable broaching the subject with your doctor. Generally, the situations in which patients explore options outside of biomedicine are those in which the patient is not improving. In cases where the problem is acute, Western treatment options usually solve things quickly. For patients with chronic conditions, healing may be slower and require greater effort on the part of the patient and the physician. Often both parties become frustrated with what appears to be a lack of progress. Eastern medicine is well suited to treating people in such circumstances. As we have mentioned previously, some patients do worry that their doctor would be offended at the suggestion of a complementary therapy, but in truth, that rarely happens. In our experience, most Western practitioners are interested only in their patients' well-being and are delighted at the prospect of successful treatment through Eastern medicine.

Occasionally, in difficult cases where a patient has not improved with conventional treatments, a physician may feel a sense of failure or embarrassment that she has not been able to help that person sufficiently. Following an honest and respectful discussion of Western and Eastern treatment options, doctors and patients alike are often relieved that a new plan has been formulated. Although the Western physician may not be administering the Eastern treatment herself, she would still be a part of your healthcare team and would certainly do her best to facilitate this new aspect of your care where possible.

Finally, it is very important that you keep your doctor aware of any non-allopathic treatments that you are undergoing. Even if you have decided on your own to seek the help of an Eastern medical practitioner, your Western doctor needs to know this, particularly if you are taking any herbs or supplements. Many medications can interact with herbs, supplements, and foods, leading to dangerous situations in which the action of the drug is either accentuated or diminished, resulting in medical complications.

Keep in mind that acupuncture and herbs, while extraordinarily effective, are not the only components of Eastern medicine. Acupuncture and herbs are treatments that are given to you by a skilled professional. But healthy food, moderate exercise, and a quiet mind are the foundation of Eastern medicine, as well as many other healing traditions. Although both your Western and Eastern healthcare providers can offer you encouragement and effective strategies for improving your physical and emotional well-being and sleep, only you can enact these changes to achieve optimal health.

CHAPTER 2

The Gastrointestinal System and Glucose Metabolism in Health and Disease

Understanding Our Digestive System

Every day we are bombarded by information about the latest "super food," supplement, or nutraceutical that promises us better health and longer life. We are reminded to choose organic produce whenever possible, and arguments abound regarding the "best" diet to follow. But no matter how nutrient-dense the food you eat, you will not receive the benefits if you cannot digest it.

A properly functioning digestive system is of paramount importance. The digestive system encompasses the gastrointestinal tract (including the mouth, esophagus, stomach, and small and large intestines), liver, gallbladder, and pancreas. These organs function together to break down food then absorb the useable portions to be utilized for growth, cell repair, and energy. The process of using energy for these activities of living is called metabolism. The waste products of digestion and metabolism are removed from the body by various organ systems. The digestive system removes the solid waste. The kidneys and bladder remove the liquid waste, and the lungs remove the carbon dioxide that results from the biochemical processes that produce energy.

This is a very complicated process and each component needs to work effectively. Even people who have access to high quality food will become malnourished if their digestive system is unable to extract and absorb the nutrients within. A body that is malnourished will inevitably develop disease. These diseases may stem from increased susceptibility to viruses and bacteria due to a weakened immune system or from a gradual breakdown of the normal physiological processes that keep us functioning. Disordered physiologic processes that are linked to problems within the gastrointestinal system include metabolic conditions such as diabetes and obesity. There is a lot of overlap in the pathophysiology of gastrointestinal disorders, obesity, and diabetes. Some people suffer from all three conditions. The numbers are staggering.

In 2012, an estimated seventy million Americans suffered from gastrointestinal disorders. Illness that arises from these conditions can cause a wide variety of symptoms and can lead to decreased quality of life. The resulting ambulatory care visits, hospitalizations, procedures, and indirect costs such as missed work tallied $142 billion.[1] According to the 2018 update, these statistics have not improved and represent a higher expenditure than for many other diagnostic categories; for example, heart disease ($113 billion).[2]

As of 2016, ninety-three million Americans were obese as measured by their body mass index, and the rates of obesity are accelerating.[3] Over the next three decades, unless this trend is reversed, Americans' life expectancy will be shortened by almost four years because of medical conditions related to obesity such as heart disease and diabetes. Also, during the same time frame, the United States is expected to spend over 13 percent of the total funds allotted to healthcare each year treating the consequences of obesity. This was the highest expected annual expenditure used for

---

1. Anne F. Peery, MD, et al. "Burden of Gastrointestinal Disease in the United States: 2012 Update," *Gastroenterology* 143, no. 5 (Nov. 2012): 1179–1187e3, https://doi.org/10.1053/j.gastro.2012.08.002.

2. Anne F. Peery, MD, et al. "Burden and Cost of Gastrointestinal, Liver, and Pancreatic Diseases in the United States: 2018 Update," *Gastroenterology* 156, no. 1 (2019): 254–272.

3. Craig M. Hales, MD, et al. "Prevalence of Obesity Among Adults and Youth: United States, 2015–2016," NCHS Data Brief No. 288, Oct. 2017, https://www.cdc.gov/nchs/data/databriefs/db288.pdf.

obesity related illnesses of the fifty-five countries surveyed in the Organization for Economic Cooperation and Development's 2019 report.[4]

Diabetes and prediabetes affected twenty-three million and eighty-four million Americans, respectively, in 2017.[5] It is estimated that another seven million people have diabetes but remain undiagnosed. The cost of caring for only the twenty-three million Americans known to have diabetes is more than $245 billion.[6]

So, about one in five Americans is affected by a digestive disorder, almost one in three is obese, and one in three suffers from diabetes or prediabetes (some people may have to contend with all three conditions). That one person might be you or someone in your immediate family. Chances are you have experienced some of the direct and indirect costs.

Because the gastrointestinal and metabolic system is so complex, many things can go wrong with any of the organs involved in the digestive process. In fact, the National Institute of Diabetes and Digestive and Kidney Diseases gives information about forty different digestive problems alone on their website. Also included are pages covering diabetes, prediabetes, and weight management.[7]

The discussion and general recommendations that follow may be useful to anyone struggling with any digestive disorder, diabetes, or obesity, but you should still talk to your healthcare provider regarding the specifics of diagnosis and treatment. As we shall see, gastrointestinal and metabolic disease has many causes and affects all the other organ systems in the body. To begin unraveling this complex process, let's start with some

---

4. Organization for Economic Co-operation and Development, "Heavy Burden of Obesity: A Quick Guide for Policy Makers," https://www.oecd.org/health/health-systems/Heavy-burden-of-obesity-Policy-Brief-2019.pdf

5. Centers for Disease Control and Prevention, National Diabetes Statistics Report, 2017 (Atlanta, GA: Centers for Disease Control and Prevention, US Department of Health and Human Services, 2017), https://www.cdc.gov/diabetes/data/statistics/statistics-report.html.

6. American Diabetes Association, "Economic Costs of Diabetes in the U.S. in 2012," *Diabetes Care* 36, no. 4 (2013):1033–1046, https://doi.org/10.2337/dc12-2625.

7. National Institute of Diabetes and Digestive and Kidney Diseases, "Digestive Diseases," https://www.niddk.nih.gov/health-information/digestive-diseases, accessed July 4, 2017 and January 1, 2020.

anatomy and physiology; that is, what constitutes your gastrointestinal and metabolic system and how it works.

The Anatomy of the Digestive System

In order to understand digestive illness, we must understand our digestive system and how it performs its functions to keep the body well nourished.

Your digestive system is made up of the hollow organs of the gastrointestinal tract (GI tract), plus the liver, pancreas, and gallbladder. The hollow organs of the GI tract are the mouth, esophagus, stomach, small intestine, large intestine, and anus. The liver and pancreas are solid. The gallbladder is actually hollow, but is not attached end-to-end to the hollow tubes like the intestines, so it falls into its own category.

First, so you understand the roadmap of your GI tract, we will outline the route your food takes from the beginning to the end of the GI tract. We will discuss the biochemical process of digestion in a moment. After food enters your mouth, you chew and swallow it. It then travels down your esophagus into your stomach. From the stomach, the food passes into your small intestine. The small intestine is divided into three parts based on its structure and function. The first part is the duodenum, the jejunum is the middle portion, and the ileum is the third part that connects to the large intestine. The large intestine consists of the appendix, cecum, colon, and rectum. The appendix is a slender pouch about the size of your little finger that is attached to the cecum. The cecum is the first part of the large intestine. The colon, which has three portions, is next. Imagine the colon like a three-sided box outlining the perimeter of your abdomen. The ascending colon starts at the lower right corner and goes up to upper right, near your liver. The transverse colon is draped across the top or abdomen, under your diaphragm. Your descending colon runs from the left upper corner of your abdomen, near your spleen, down to your rectum. The rectum is the end of the large intestine, where the waste is expelled. The anus is the muscular ring that controls the exit of stool from the rectum. From beginning to end, your GI tract measures over thirty feet when unraveled.

The Function of the Digestive System

Your digestive system is designed to take the food you eat and break it down into its component parts called nutrients. There are different types

The Anatomy of the Gastrointestinal Tract

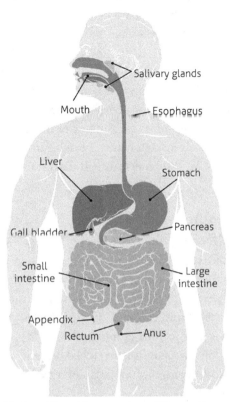

Illustration by Christos Georghiou, courtesy of Dreamstime.

of nutrients that are absorbed into your bloodstream and act as building blocks within your body to support growth and cell repair. Some nutrients are broken down further to supply the energy you need to simply live and breathe. You need all the different nutrient groups to stay healthy—proteins, fats, carbohydrates, vitamins, minerals, and water. The larger nutrient molecules undergo various processes and are broken down even further. Proteins are turned into amino acids, fats are broken down to fatty acids and glycerol, and carbohydrates are broken down to simple sugars. Once foods are broken into sufficiently small fragments, your body can absorb them for use in various parts of the body.

Nerves, hormones, and the bacteria that live in your gut have a tremendous influence on this process and the health of your GI tract. This, in turn, determines the health of your entire body, including your brain and emotional well-being. Examining the process of digestion is a bit like listening to a concert. Whether you are listening to a classical string quartet or a heavy metal band, each musician has an individual part to play. The notes may be different, but the intent and timing are the same. The musical piece starts at one instant in time and all the players work synchronously to the end. Like musicians, various systems must work together seamlessly for your food to be properly digested. These aspects are mechanical, biochemical, neurological, and hormonal. Both human cells and bacteria are deeply involved. But, before we delve into these intricate components of the digestive system, let's finish discussing the mechanical aspect of digestion.

The Mechanical Aspect of Digestion

Above, we talked about the different parts of the digestive system through which your food must pass in order to be absorbed into your body. So how does the food get from one end of this thirty-foot tract to the other? The first part is fairly obvious. You chew your food and then swallow as your tongue pushes the food into the back of your throat. After it leaves your mouth, your food is now in your esophagus. At this point, your brain becomes aware that your esophagus is stretched out and sends signals to the esophageal muscles to contract in a particular fashion. This contraction pattern is called peristalsis.

Peristalsis is the process by which the muscular walls of the GI tract contract and move your food through your digestive system. The muscles behind the mass of food you've chewed and swallowed (called the bolus) get tight and push the food along the GI tract. Imagine squeezing toothpaste from the back of the tube to the tip and you will get the idea. At the same time, the muscles of the GI tract in front of your food relax so that the food can move forward. The process of peristalsis is also responsible for the mixing of your food to break it down mechanically. Peristalsis is an automatic process, controlled by the parasympathetic branch of the autonomic nervous system. We will talk much more about how your nervous system affects your digestion shortly.

Once the peristaltic action of your esophagus pushes the food down to the lower end, the muscular ring that separates the esophagus and stomach relaxes, allowing the food to pass into your stomach. This muscular ring is called the esophageal sphincter. When the bolus of food has completely passed through the esophageal sphincter, it closes to prohibit food from moving back up into the esophagus.

While in the stomach, your food is mixed with digestive juices. This slurry of food and digestive juices is called "chyme." Your food reaches the consistency of chyme through the movement of muscles of the stomach wall, which are very strong. If you have ever felt like your stomach was churning, you were right!

From the stomach, the chyme passes through another sphincter to reach the first part of the small intestine, the duodenum. Here, the chyme is exposed to components of the body's digestive juices from the pancreas and the liver. Digestive enzymes from the pancreas and bile from the liver that is stored in the gallbladder all join together via a system of ducts. The smaller ducts flow into larger ones until they finally amalgamate into one duct that empties into the duodenum. The duodenum itself also secretes enzymes and hormones that regulate peristalsis and mechanical processing of the chyme. We will be discussing this biochemical aspect of digestion in the next section.

As your food travels through the remainder of the small intestine via the process of peristalsis, nutrients and water are absorbed into your bloodstream through the wall of the small intestine. This process of absorption is intricate, and its disruption may be the cause of many chronic illnesses, as we shall see. Once in the veins of the intestines, the nutrients are carried to the liver where they undergo processing before being sent to the heart and pumped out to the rest of your body.

What remains of your food enters your large intestine. It is considered a waste product, but even at this stage, water is absorbed and some undigested food is further broken down by bacteria. This allows you to access more energy and nutrients. With most of the water removed, this waste product becomes stool. Finally, the muscular contractions of peristalsis move the stool into your rectum, where it is kept until you have a bowel movement, pushing it out and completing the process.

The Biochemical Aspect of Digestion

Let's start back at the top.

As you chew, your salivary glands release saliva that moistens your food. Saliva also contains several enzymes that start the digestive process before your food even gets to your stomach. These enzymes are called amylase, lingual lipase, kallikrein, and lysozyme. Amylase begins the process of digestion of starches and lingual lipase starts the process of digestion of fats. Kallikrein is a compound that helps to break down proteins into smaller units. Lysozyme does not actually participate in the digestion of your food. Rather, it helps to protect you against dangerous bacteria by breaking down their cell walls. This allows water to enter the bacteria. The bacteria then swell and burst. This process is called "lysis," which explains how lysozyme was named.

No new biochemical components are added to your food while it is in the esophagus, but once it arrives in the stomach new compounds are mixed in. There are various types of cells located in the lining of the stomach, each with its own task. Some secrete another form of lipase called gastric lipase that further breaks down fats. Other cells secrete pepsinogen, an inactive form of the digestive enzyme pepsin that helps digest proteins. Pepsinogen is changed into pepsin when it comes in contact with stomach acid (hydrochloric acid) that is released by yet another type of cell. Hydrochloric acid also destroys dangerous bacteria and viruses.

While stomach acid is essential to digestion, the stomach lining needs a way to protect itself so the very acid it secretes does not damage it. This defense comes in the form of mucin, a gel-like substance that is produced in the stomach and guards the cell lining there and all along the intestinal tract. Two other compounds produced in the stomach are intrinsic factor (IF) and gastrin. Intrinsic factor binds to vitamin B12 to protect it against the stomach acid, keeping it safe until it can be absorbed in the last portion of the small intestine, the ileum. Gastrin is a hormone that is secreted when the stomach is stretched from the food you have eaten. Gastrin essentially notifies the cells that secrete hydrochloric acid and intrinsic factor to start production.

Now the chyme is emptied into the first part of the small intestine, the duodenum. Here, more enzymes are added to the mix from both the lining of the duodenum and the pancreas to further break down your food.

Depending upon whether your meal contained mostly fats, carbohydrates, or proteins, the duodenum and pancreas adjust the kinds of enzymes that are released to ensure optimal digestion. Bile that is created in the liver and stored in the gallbladder is also released into the duodenum to emulsify the fats in your food and allow easier digestion. This is like adding extra dish soap when you are scrubbing a greasy pot. The detergent surrounds the fat molecules and makes it simpler to break down. This is exactly how bile aids in the digestion of dietary fat.

Hormones are also released in the duodenum and pancreas. In response to the acidity of the chyme from the stomach, the duodenum produces a hormone called secretin that tells the pancreas to release its enzymes and also produce bicarbonate to buffer the acidity of the chyme. Secretin also slows down gastrin production by the stomach. Another very interesting hormone that is produced in the duodenum is cholecystokinin (CCK). CCK acts as both a hormone and a neurotransmitter, an attribute we will discuss in the next section. As a digestive hormone, CCK increases gallbladder contractions so that bile will flow into the duodenum. CCK also initiates the release of pancreatic enzymes and bicarbonate. The most important hormones created by the pancreas are insulin and glucagon. This pair of hormones works together to maintain normal glucose levels in your blood. Insulin allows the cells in your body to absorb and utilize glucose, drawing the glucose out of your bloodstream and keeping your glucose (blood sugar) levels from getting too high. Conversely, glucagon is released when your blood sugar levels are getting too low or your body senses the impending need for extra energy. Glucagon will then stimulate the cells that store glucose to release it into your bloodstream, making it available for immediate use. Disruptions in the balance and utilization of insulin and glucagon can lead to serious illness, as we shall see.

Throughout the small and large intestine, the inner surface is lined with cells called enterocytes. These cells absorb nutrients, water, salts, and vitamins, but they also secrete a hormone called leptin. Leptin, which is also secreted by your fat cells, tells your brain that you are full. It is also known as the satiety hormone. Leptin's counterpart is called ghrelin and this hormone tells your brain that you are hungry. Ghrelin is secreted primarily in the stomach and small intestine. Disturbances in the production and processing of these two hormones have dire consequences for our metabolism. We will be discussing more about the leptin/ghrelin balance in chapter 5.

Now, having examined the mechanical and biochemical processes involved in digestion, let's look at the way your nervous system is involved.

The Neurological Aspect of Digestion

Before a single morsel of food passes your lips, your nervous system is preparing your body to eat. Simply the sight of food, the smell, and even the sound of it cooking is enough to start the secretion of saliva and gastric juices. The sensory input of your eyes, nose, and ears stimulate your brain. Your brain then sends signals to your gastrointestinal tract via the vagus nerve to start the digestive process. But, your brain is not the only part of your nervous system that governs the functioning of your GI tract. There is a distinct branch of your autonomic nervous system that focuses entirely on digestion and metabolism. This branch is called the enteric nervous system (ENS).

The ENS contains fifty million to one hundred million nerve cells. This is as many as are found in your spinal cord.[8] When food distends the walls of your GI tract, the nerves of your ENS coordinate digestion by stimulating the production of digestive juices and calibrating the speed with which your meal transits through your gut. Your ENS will allow more time for steak to be digested than it will for tofu, for example. The ENS controls the muscular contraction and relaxation of your intestinal walls, sending your food along the GI tract at the appropriate time based on its nutritional make up. The ENS is even responsible for the timing of the migrating motor complex, which is a strong, slow wave of muscular contractions that occur every ninety minutes when there is no food in your intestines. This pressure wave sweeps out the debris of your GI tract, from undigested bits of food to unwanted microbes. All these actions occur under the direction of the ENS with minimal input from the central nervous system in the brain. The ENS even contains large amounts of the neurotransmitter called serotonin. In fact, 95 percent of the serotonin

---

8. Emeran Mayer, MD, *The Mind-Gut Connection: How the Hidden Conversation within Our Bodies Impacts Our Mood, Our Choices, and Our Overall Health*, (New York: Harper Wave, 2016), 11.

found in the body is located in cells associated with the ENS.[9] Serotonin is a signaling molecule that most of us think only relates to psychological well-being. In fact, serotonin is vital for normal gut motility and appetite as well as for sleep, pain sensitivity, and mood. The complexity of the ENS and its serotonin system led Michael Gershon, cell biologist and ground-breaking gut researcher, to dub the ENS the "second brain."

Not only does the brain in your gut operate virtually independently, it sends information up to the brain in your skull. The two are in constant communication via the vagus nerve and hormonal and inflammatory signaling molecules. Renowned gastroenterologist and expert in brain-gut communication, Dr. Emeran Mayer, views the gut as a "vast sensory organ" that contains enough tiny receptors to cover an area the size of a basketball court.[10] Dr. Mayer notes that gut signals sent to the brain can generate awareness of gut sensations, both pleasant and unpleasant. For example, you may experience a sensation of fullness after a delightful meal with friends or nausea after eating fish that has spoiled. All sensations, such calm well-being or butterflies in your stomach before a performance, are registered and recorded. Your brain, in turn, sends signals to your gut that create gut reactions. These sensations and responses are stored in your memory and can influence your decisions and behavior in the future. A basic example would be deciding not to eat fish that has a pungent smell. A more nuanced example would be the way we use our gut intuition to make important decisions, such as who to marry. In his book, *The Mind-Gut Connection*, Dr. Mayer draws a comparison between this bidirectional communication between the gut and the brain and the concept of yin and yang.

> *In Chinese philosophy, the concept of yin and yang describes how opposite or contrary forces can be viewed as complementary and interconnected, and how they give rise to a unifying whole by interacting with each other. When applied to the brain-gut axis, we can view our gut feelings as the yin, and gut reactions as the yang. Just as yin and yang are the two complementary principles of the same entity—the brain-gut connection—both the feelings and the reactions are different aspects of the same bidirectional brain-gut*

---

9. Mayer, *The Mind-Gut Connection*, 12.
10. Mayer, 12.

network that plays such a crucial role in our well-being, our emo-
tions, and our ability to make intuitive decisions.[11]

One can also see similarities between the bidirectional gut-brain communication that is mediated by the vagus nerve and the connection between the dan tian via the penetrating vessel, one of the eight extraordinary channels. Millenia ago, the Chinese described these pathways that allowed communication and balance between the body and the mind.

The ability of your brain to connect sensory input from gut to the emotional response that it generates is hardwired. This capability confers a survival advantage in that it helps us to make decisions that are usually in our best interest. Sometimes, however, our life experiences sensitize the both the gut and the brain resulting in disproportionate emotional and physical responses to stimuli that are perceived as dangerous. Imagine going through any traumatic event. Over time, the body's reaction to this stress settles down, but in some people the nervous system remains on high alert leading to exaggerated responses to events or situations that are similar to the initiating trauma. This is true in both brains. In the ENS, alterations in gut function and the composition of the gut bacteria play a significant role in GI disorders such as IBS, as well as anxiety disorders and depression.[12] Moreover, people who experience trauma in early childhood are more likely to suffer from these interrelated conditions.[13] Those with anxiety disorders tend also to have problems with chronic diarrhea and those with depression tend to be constipated. Both conditions are generally accompanied by abdominal pain. Even people whose mothers experience severe stress and trauma are at higher risk for stress-sensitive conditions like gut disorders, psychoemotional problems, and obesity. This propensity can be passed down genetically for generations.[14]

Why would this happen? How could a genetic predisposition toward an exaggerated stress response possibly be of benefit? If you think about this from an evolutionary point of view, it makes perfect sense. If a mother (of any species) lives in what she perceives as a dangerous

---

11. Mayer, 14.
12. Mayer, 43.
13. Mayer, 45.
14. Mayer, 130.

environment, the ability to confer a heightened sense of alertness and a rapidly activated fight-or-flight response would be a survival advantage to her offspring. Even though she is unaware of the process, the mother is able to pass on these traits genetically at conception and also at birth by an alteration in her vaginal bacteria that then programs the infant's gastrointestinal bacteria. During early childhood, these traits may be reinforced through behavioral cues. This heightened fight-or-flight response becomes problematic when we live in comparatively safe environments.

Fortunately, as humans, we can identify and understand this mismatch between normal stressors and exaggerated responses. Our brains are able to reason and are capable of controlling these reactions. We can learn to override our automatic heightened responses to stressors and learn new ways of behaving when our fight-and-flight response is triggered. Techniques that help us rewire our brains and emotional circuitry include cognitive behavioral therapy and mind-body interventions that reduce stress such as meditation and qigong. Not only can these techniques ease emotional discomfort, but physical symptoms such as abdominal pain and bowel dysfunction can also be relieved. Of course, there are medications and supplements that can be employed which we will discuss in later chapters.

We have seen that there are many facets of the digestive system: mechanical, biochemical, and neurological. Now we will discuss perhaps the most fascinating component of all, the biological part of the digestive system that is *within* us, but not *of* us—the microbiome.

The Human Microbiome

Ever since the first microbes were viewed through a light microscope in 1632, our understanding of these single-celled creatures has continued to evolve. Over the centuries, our perception of bacteria has shifted. Initially, we looked at all bacteria as the enemy—the cause of life-threatening diseases that should be eradicated. But over the last several decades we have come to appreciate the intricate web that these organisms have spun.

The entire world is covered with microbes. They were here billions of years before us and are responsible for the creation of earth's ecosystem. Dr. Martin Blaser, director of the Human Microbiome Project at NYU and author of *Missing Microbes*, poetically describes how bacteria drove the chemical reactions that form our biosphere.

> *Slowly, inexorably, through trial and error across the deepness of time, they invented the complex and robust feedback systems that to this day support all life on Earth.*[15]

Bacteria have been found in the land, sea, and sky. They have been discovered in volcanic rock, glaciers, and soil worldwide. In the oceans, they have been isolated from the deepest caverns in the Marianas Trench and on floating plastic on the surface where they digest our debris. In the atmosphere, they contribute to the formation of cirrus clouds and snow, as well as the decontamination of pollution.[16] Microbes make life on Earth possible. They decompose dead organic matter and fortify the soil. They are key to many biochemical processes from brewing beer to bioengineering.

Not only are bacteria all around us, they are in us, too—us and every other living creature on Earth. All animals have their own set of microbes, unique to their species, which have coevolved over millennia.[17] The host and the microbes have formed a mutually beneficial relationship, each sustaining the other in many different ways. This relationship is called "symbiosis." There are estimated to be more than one hundred trillion cells in the human microbiome. Contrast this to the number of cells in the human body: thirty trillion. This means that of all the cells encased in and on your body, 70 to 90 percent of them are nonhuman.[18] The microbiome is estimated to weigh approximately three pounds—about as much as your brain. Some researchers feel the microbiome should be classified as an organ unto itself. There are groups of symbiotic bacteria on your skin, up your nose, in your ears, and, of course, in every part of your digestive system. So, what are they all doing there?

The microbiome of your gut, which is the focus of this section, is responsible for a vast array of biochemical processes that keep you alive and

---

15. Martin J. Blaser, MD, *Missing Microbes*, (Henry Holt and Company: New York, 2018), 13.

16. Blaser, 17.

17. Blaser, 23.

18. Blaser, Missing Microbes, 25.

in good health. These responsibilities include absorption of nutrients, training the immune system, keeping harmful bacteria in check, producing vitamin K that helps your blood clot, metabolizing certain drugs, digesting particular starches, signaling hunger and fullness, and producing neurotransmitters that affect your emotional health.

For the most part, we live in harmony with our microbiome, but you can see that with so many processes dependent on these gut bacteria, a lot can go wrong if the there is an imbalance. Dr. Blaser and other researchers have noted a shift in the composition of the human microbiome over the decades. In *Missing Microbes*, Dr. Blaser expounds upon his theory. He contends that it is the loss of diversity within the human microbiome that has led to this epidemic of gastrointestinal diseases as well as many other related conditions such as asthma, autoimmune disease, depression, allergies, obesity, and dementia.

Some causes of gut microbiome disruption include lack of exposure to beneficial bacteria as we obsess with hygiene and cleanliness, overuse of antibiotics for non-life-threatening illnesses, increased rate of cesarean section that deprives the infant of exposure to the mother's vaginal microbiome, and decreased rates and length of breastfeeding. These issues are responsible for a profound shift in the human microbiome such that key bacteria are being lost. The other bacteria in the microbiome depend upon these key players to perform certain biochemical reactions needed for optimal functioning of the rest of the microbes. Dr. Blaser's research reveals the science behind these factors and the concomitant rise of these chronic diseases. An in-depth discussion can be found in *Missing Microbes* and is highly recommended.

Certain health conditions are associated with certain microbial profiles. For example, more than 90 percent of the bacteria in the colon are of two types, Firmicutes and Bacteroidetes. The relative proportions of these two types of bacteria can determine your risk for disease. People who have elevated levels Firmicutes and lower levels of Bacteroidetes in their colon tend to be obese. The reverse is true for people who are lean. The reason for this is that the Firmicutes bacteria are expert at extracting more calories from food that can then be absorbed in the colon. The ability to obtain additional calories from less food would have been quite an advantage in times of scarcity, but in our society of overabundance, it is a liability. Not only does this microbial profile lead to obesity, it increases your risk for diabetes and heart disease.[19]

While we each have a unique microbial fingerprint, there is overlap in the metabolites that various bacteria produce so that we can adapt to different diets depending upon the availability of food sources. This is why humans the world over can survive on wildly different diets, from entirely vegan to entirely animal based. We will talk about what foods your gut microbes prefer and which foods will lead to the production of the most healthful metabolites, but the population and demographics of your microbiome do not change significantly with dietary modifications.[20]

How the microbiome influences your health for better or worse depends on many factors. One factor that is definitely within your control is what you eat. For years we thought that eating significant amounts of insoluble dietary fiber was only useful to keep your bowels moving regularly. Now we know that certain bacteria in your colon can process fiber that we, ourselves, cannot digest. They then produce short chain fatty acids, which are a type of molecule that contains less than six carbon atoms. There are several different types of short chain fatty acids (SCFAs), and they all have beneficial healing properties. Overall, SFCAs help to control appetite, regulate metabolism and body fat, optimize immune function, and improve emotional well-being.[21] In turn, these changes help decrease your risk for diabetes, obesity, heart disease, autoimmune conditions, and mental health problems. Diets high in insoluble fiber may decrease your risk for certain cancers and SFCAs may be the key reason.[22] Much depends on the types of bacteria that make up your microbiome and how strongly the beneficial bacteria are represented in the whole system. You can encourage the health of these beneficial microbes through diet modification, which we will discuss further in the coming chapters.

---

19. H. Kumar, et al. "Gut Microbiota as an Epigenetic Regulator: Pilot Study Based on Whole-Genome Methylation Analysis", *mBio*, DOI: 10.1128/mBio.02113-14.

20. Mayer, *The Mind-Gut Connection*, 217.

21. Michael Greger, MD, *How Not to Diet* (New York: Flatiron Books, 2019), 122.

22. Dallas R. Donohoe et al, "A Gnotobiotic Mouse Model Demonstrates That Dietary Fiber Protects against Colorectal Tumorigenesis in a Microbiota- and Butyrate-Dependent Manner," *Cancer Discovery* 4, no.12 (Dec. 2014): 1387–1397, https://doi.org/10.1158/2159-8290.CD-14-0501.

In recent years there has been an explosion of research into the function of the microbiome and how it interacts with our neurological system through the enteric nervous system in the GI tract. We have already talked about the importance of this "second brain." Clearly the microbiome influences our health and well-being, but there are also remarkable examples of how microbes can influence the actual behavior and decision-making of the host.

The parasite *Toxoplasma gondii* is a prime example of how microorganisms can target specific brain structures to influence host behaviors. *T. gondii* can infect all species but can only reproduce within the intestines of cats. The cysts (essentially *T. gondii* offspring) that result are excreted in the cat's stool. Once the cyst reaches mature form, it needs to get back into a cat in order to reproduce. The way it does this is nothing short of ingenious. When a rat or mouse comes along and eats the cat excrement, the *T. gondii* infects the rodent and targets its brain. It alters specific areas of the brain so that the rodent no longer fears cats but is actually attracted to the smell of cat urine. Furthermore, *T. gondii* slows down the rodent's muscle coordination and response so that it is much more likely to be caught and eaten! In studies that have been performed in *T. gondii*-infected humans, a similar decrease in motor coordination seems to be prevalent and is associated with an increased rate of accidental injuries.[23]

Generally, the organisms of our microbiome are helpful, not harmful. The relationship between our gut bacteria and us is symbiotic, meaning that it is mutually beneficial. We know that single-celled microbes predated multicellular creatures by billions of years and were, of course, metabolically active. Some of these metabolites were signaling molecules that are similar to the hormones and neurotransmitters that are present in the enteric nervous system of our guts. About five hundred million years ago, some microbes started living inside newly evolved multicellular creatures, supplying these animals with metabolites that they could not make for themselves. Eventually, as multicellular creatures became more complex, they incorporated genetic information from their microbes, allowing the

---

23. J. Flegr, "Influence of Latent Toxoplasma Infection on Human Personality, Physiology, and Morphology: Pros and Cons of the Toxoplasma-Human Model in Studying the Manipulation Hypothesis," *Journal of Experimental Biology* 216 (2013): 127–133, https:// doi.org/10.1242/jeb.073635.

development of the enteric nervous system.[24] Even today, our microbiome makes up about 40 percent of the metabolites found in our bloodstream.[25] The signaling molecules that are elaborated by our gut bacteria are equivalent to our hormones and neurotransmitters and could be considered a shared language.

Dr. Blaser, Dr. Mayer, and other scientists contend that knowledge of the ways the gut, microbiome, and brain interact require us to change the way we view our physiology. We strongly agree. We can no longer apply the reductionist view that our bodies are machines and we are simply the sum of our parts. We must acknowledge that our existence is the result of a complicated, interdependent group of systems. We cannot wreak havoc on one aspect of this web without consequence to others. If we ignore the health of our gut-brain-microbiome axis we are essentially ignoring the health of our entire body, mind, and spirit.

Throughout the remainder of this book we will discuss the connection between your gut microbiome, your brain, and your well-being; how to feed your microbiome to achieve an ideal balance of bacteria; and how the ancient practices of meditation and qigong can influence the health the microbiome.

How Chronic Inflammation Affects Digestion and Metabolism

First, from a Western perspective, let's look at the biology of chronic disease. At first glance, there may not seem to be a link between all the chronic illnesses that plague us. Certainly, diabetes, heart disease, hypertension, and obesity are often seen together, but what about the others? Digestive disorders, chronic pain, arthritis, Alzheimer's, asthma, depression? It may not be obvious, but there is a common thread. Disruption of cellular function on a molecular level can be due to chronic inflammation, oxidative stress (the by-product of biochemical processes within the cell), and short-

---

24. Mayer, *The Mind-Gut Connection*, 91.
25. Mayer, 100.

Serotonin

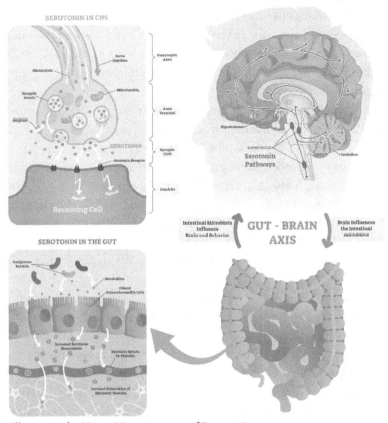

Illustration by VectorMine, courtesy of Dreamstime.

ened telomeres.[26] Telomeres are noncoding DNA sequences that are found at the ends of each chromosome. The telomeres protect the coding DNA from damage during cell replication. Telomeres and their associated enzyme, telomerase, were discovered in the 1980s by Drs. Elizabeth Blackburn, Carol Greider, and Jack Szostak, who share a Nobel Prize for their groundbreaking work. Dr. Blackburn likens the telomere to the plastic bits on the ends of your shoelaces that prevent the shoelace from fraying. Dur-

---

26. Clara Correia-Melo, Graeme Hewitt, and Joao F Passos, "Telomeres, Oxidative Stress, and Inflammatory Factors: Partners in Cellular Senescence?" *Longev Healthspan* 3 no. 1 (2014), https://doi.org/10.1186/2046-2395-3-1.

ing each chromosome replication, the telomere shortens and then is rebuilt by telomerase. This is how telomeres protect the essential information within your cells, and it seems that the longer your telomeres, the greater the buffer you have against cell death. Chronic inflammation leads to oxidative stress and telomere shortening. Soon, the damage is too great, and the cell cannot recover. At that point, the cell initiates a "self-destruct program" called apoptosis.

Inflammation in and of itself is not a bad thing. In fact, inflammation is a critical process in healing. It is the body's normal response to acute injury or infection. If you scrape your knee or catch pneumonia, white cells within your blood release certain chemicals. These are called inflammatory markers. These markers tell your body to increase blood circulation to the affected area. Your knee, for instance, will start to look redder and feel warmer following the injury. These are signs that your immune system is responding correctly. The greater blood circulation will bring more nutrients and infection-fighting cells to the damaged part of your body.

If you could not mount a proper immune response, you would die. You would succumb to the first viral or bacterial infection that came along. However, it seems that something has gone awry on a very large scale. It has been discovered that constant low-grade inflammation contributes significantly to chronic disease because the immune system starts to attack normal tissue throughout the body. Your gut is particularly vulnerable to chronic inflammation. Continual low-grade inflammation in the GI tract may set off a series of events that leads to wide spread inflammation affecting many organ systems. This sort of inflammation, dubbed "meta-inflammation"[27] or "whole-body inflammation,"[28] is not a response to acute injury or infection but rather is induced by our lifestyle habits. While it is true that environmental toxins can also cause inflammation, we can still reduce our risk for chronic disease by making better decisions. Our choices surrounding food, alcohol, cigarettes, exercise, sleep, and stress management heavily influence our immune systems. By continually

---

27. Wendy Kohatsu, MD, "The Anti-Inflammatory Diet," in *Integrative Medicine*, 3rd ed., ed. David Rakel, MD (Philadelphia: Saunders, Elsevier, 2012), 2297.

28. Andrew Weil, MD, "Ask Dr. Weil," http://www.drweil.com/drw/u/QAA401013/Reducing-Whole-Body-Inflammation.html, accessed Jan 28, 2014.

making poor choices, we overwhelm our bodies. In computer parlance, there is a saying: "Garbage in, garbage out." From a Western perspective, chronic disease is the logical result of long-term input that promotes inflammation and tissue damage.

Eastern medicine looks at chronic illness in much the same way. As we discussed in the first chapter of this book, good health is regarded as a natural consequence of balanced living. Blood and qi flow easily through all the channels of the body. Essence, energy, and spirit are in harmony. All this is primarily achieved through moderate diet, exercise, sleep, and meditative practices. While acupuncture and herbs figure prominently in Eastern medicine, it is adherence to a healthful regimen that is the cornerstone of this healing system.

When your diet is poor, when you do not get enough sleep and exercise, or when you are under stress, your body becomes vulnerable, slightly weakened, and energetically unbalanced. From an Eastern viewpoint, diseases arise because of such imbalances. These disturbances can have an external or internal source and could involve not only the body but the mind and the spirit as well. The symptoms may be subtle, at least from the point of view of a Western practitioner who may not be trained to elicit or acknowledge these indicators of impending disease.

One of the strengths of Eastern medicine is the recognition that particular patterns of symptoms and signs may indicate imbalance. If left uncorrected, these energetic dysfunctions will lead to disturbances of qi and blood circulation and ultimately organ disharmony. In using the word "organ" we are referring to not only the anatomic structure of an organ, but its physiology, its function, and its areas of influence throughout the body. In Eastern medicine, nothing exists in isolation. A disturbance in one channel or organ will affect all the others. This is an elegant explanation of the neurological, immune, and endocrine systems at work. As we are have already seen, your gut and metabolic health is dependent upon these systems functioning harmoniously. After so many years of trying to reduce the human body to the smallest component, cutting edge science is bearing out the concept that the intricate interplay between larger systems determines a person's state of health.

Now, you are probably asking, "Can anything be done to reverse this epidemic of chronic inflammation and subsequent illness?" What with all the chemicals in our water and air, all the unhealthy additives inserted into processed food, and all the stressors of modern life, good health seems like a lost cause. But you *can* take control of your own well-being. Decreasing inflammation in the GI tract is imperative for decreasing inflammation in all other organ systems.

Throughout this book we will teach you different ways to decrease inflammation, but the best and first step is to eat more plants. Even if this is the only change you make, your health will improve significantly. If you eat a healthy diet based on plants, you could decrease your chance of developing a chronic disease by at least 60 percent.[29] You do not need to become a vegetarian, but you need to make fruits and vegetables the mainstay of your diet. More and more Western biochemical research has determined why fruits and vegetables are essential for good health. Western doctors are returning to the wisdom of their forebears, like Hippocrates, who said, "Let food be your medicine and medicine be your food."

Of course, practitioners of Eastern medicine have never forgotten this basic tenet of healthy living. They have always stressed the importance of eating plants. Why can eating plants decrease your risk for chronic disease? Because the nutrients within plants act like medications that reduce inflammation. These compounds act on specific biochemical reactions in the body and have many beneficial effects. Aside from supplying high concentrations of vitamins and minerals, plant proteins, like certain legumes, nuts, and seeds, are rich in healthy fats (omega-3 fatty acids) that have anti-inflammatory effects.

Now that you know how a plant-based diet will reduce chronic inflammation, let's take a look at other dietary and lifestyle choices you can make to reduce inflammation and optimize your health.

How the Sleep-Wake Cycle Affects the Gut

Timing is everything. Whether in a career, sports match, or international peace talks, less than perfect timing can lead to disaster.

It turns out this is also true for our health. When we sleep, when we wake, and when we eat can lay the foundation for an efficient metabolism

---

29. Wendy Kohatsu, MD, "The Anti-Inflammatory Diet," 2297.

and robust health or can set off a disastrous chain reaction that leads to chronic disease. A huge amount of research has been done on the sleep-wake cycle and its influence. From single-celled organisms to human beings, creatures as diverse as fungi and mammals experience biological cycles that repeat roughly every twenty-four hours. This daily fluctuation is called a circadian rhythm (*circa* = approximately, *dia* = day). It has been demonstrated that we humans will adopt an approximate twenty-four- to twenty-five-hour sleep-wake cycle even if we do not have any environmental cues like natural light. The part of our brain that directs this recurring cycle is the suprachiasmatic nucleus (SCN). The SCN is considered the pacemaker for the circadian rhythm. The SCN will create neurological and biochemical outputs that send instructions to other organ systems regarding how and when to function at peak performance. Circadian rhythms influence more than just when you sleep and when you wake up. The signals from the SCN also influence the fluctuations in your hormone levels, immune function, and body temperature, as well as your ability to perform physical tasks, be alert, and digest your food.

The SCN is our main circadian pacemaker and known as our "master clock" or "central clock." There is a particular gene, a version of which is found in all living creatures, that is integral to keeping this daily rhythm. This gene, known as Per, turns on and off about every twenty-four hours. Just like the intricate mechanism of a clock, there are many other genes that function together to get the Per gene to turn on and off at a regular twenty-four-hour interval. These genes are known as clock genes and any disruption in the way these genes function can lead to dysregulation of our metabolism. Clock genes are involved in other cellular functions like burning or storing glucose or fat, cell repair, and detoxification. It has been determined that almost every cell in our body contains its own circadian clock.[30] Consequently, every organ has its own circadian clock, including the gut. These clocks are called "peripheral clocks."

One of the most important environmental cues that entrain our "master clock" is blue wave light, the sort that is found in sunlight. The other significant environmental cue is food. In fact, feeding times have such a

---

30. Satchin Panda, PhD, "What Are Circadian Clocks, Where Are They, and How Can We Nurture Them?" https://blog.mycircadianclock.org/what-are-circa-dian-clocks-where-are-they-and-how-can-we-nurture-them/.

strong effect on your circadian rhythm they can actually override the entrainment effect of light. This means that your body will pay less attention to the day/night cycle if you are eating late at night when you should be going to sleep. Dr. Satchin Panda, a leading expert in circadian biology, elegantly demonstrated in rodent experiments how disrupting the daily rhythm of feeding times can lead to chronic diseases like diabetes, obesity, and fatty liver.

Dr. Panda and his research colleagues divided their cohort of mice into two groups. Both groups were given a high fat, high sugar diet, which is the rodent equivalent to human junk food. Now, like humans, mice like high fat, high sugar foods and will eat a lot of it, even getting up in the middle of the night to eat it if it is available. All creatures are basically hard-wired to prefer foods with a high caloric density and eat as much as they can when it is around. In times of scarcity, this biological imperative would improve chances of survival. When such food is abundant, however, obesity results.

Dr. Panda's mice were allowed to eat as much of this food as they wanted, but there was one difference between the groups. One group had access to food twenty-four hours a day. The other group had limited access such that they could only eat during their normal period of activity. Mice being nocturnal, they were allowed to eat at night, but the food was taken away during the day. The results of this experiment showed that, even though the calories consumed were the same in both groups, the mice that ate day and night became obese and the mice that ate at restricted times remained normal weight. Apparently, Dr. Panda was so surprised by this outcome that he repeated the study several times before he would believe the results.[31]

Next, Dr. Panda took the mice that were already obese and had diabetes, high cholesterol, and fatty liver, and restricted their feeding times to their normal period of activity. Within weeks, these mice lost 20 percent of their body fat and their diseases disappeared. These experiments were repeated with different types of mice and the results were the same.

---

31. Rangan Chatterjee, MD, Feel Better, Live More Podcast, "Why When You Eat Matters with Dr. Satchin Panda, Part 1," https://drchatterjee.com/episode-21-circadian-rhythms-and-time-restricted-feeding-with-professor-satchin-panda-part-1/.

So, are these findings reproducible in humans in real life situations? Dr. Panda wanted to determine when and what people actually eat. In order to answer this question, Dr. Panda created a study in which healthy volunteers used a smart phone application to take pictures of their food. The people in this study sent these time-stamped photos to Dr. Panda's research team who analyzed the photos, noted the times, and attributed approximate nutritional values to the food item. All personal information was scrubbed from the photo transmission so the data was anonymous and not used for commercial purposes.

Dr. Panda made several interesting discoveries. He found that the subjects ate less than 25 percent of their calories before noon and more than 35 percent of their calories after 6 p.m., indicating that a lot of people ate a substantial amount of food in the evenings when the body is less metabolically active. Dr. Panda also found that less than half of the volunteers ate their food within a fifteen-hour window. The majority of the volunteers ate their food over a fifteen-hour period *or longer* on a daily basis. The time from the first bite of food to the last seemed to parallel their waking hours. Subsequently, Dr. Panda wanted to know whether those people who ate for more than fifteen hours per day *and* were overweight could achieve the same health benefits as the obese mice through time-restricted feeding. These volunteers were asked to restrict their eating hours to a ten-hour period each day. This was the only change the volunteers were asked to make. At the end of sixteen weeks, the people in the study lost an average of four to five percent of their body fat. In a one-year follow up, most people reported maintaining the habit of time restricted eating, not due to the benefit of weight loss, but because they found they had more energy, slept better, and had less heartburn.[32]

Dr. Panda and other researchers worldwide have since demonstrated that prolonged eating duration disrupts our normal circadian rhythms. This disturbance of the central and peripheral biological clocks contributes to the development of more than one hundred chronic diseases. In the gut, the disturbance manifests in a variety of ways. Normally, when you go

---

32. S. Gill, S. Panda, "A Smartphone App Reveals Erratic Diurnal Eating Patterns in Humans That Can Be Modulated for Health Benefits," *Cell Metabolism* 22, no. 5 (Nov. 3, 2015): 789–798.

to sleep two to three hours after your last bite of food, digestion is completed. Your saliva production and intestinal function slow down at night. Every night, while you sleep approximately 10 percent of your intestinal lining is repaired. If you eat right before going to sleep, your gut is forced to process this food when it is not functioning at its peak. Dr. Panda compares this situation with workers trying to repair a highway when cars are driving along at full speed. The repairs are likely to be incomplete. When the gut does not have time to repair itself properly, damaged cells are left behind, causing inflammation. Inflammation in the lining of the GI tract is the underlying cause of many chronic gastrointestinal conditions, such as ulcerative colitis and Crohn's disease. Gut inflammation is considered a driver for diseases outside the GI tract, including obesity, depression, heart disease, and Alzheimer's.

Even your microbiome is influenced by circadian rhythms.[33] Intestinal microbe population and functional activity change throughout the day in a near twenty-four-hour cycle, which presents the gut lining with different metabolites at distinct times during the day. This influences the metabolites produced by the circadian clock genes of the gut. It seems that the body's circadian clock works synergistically with the microbial clock and the relationship is bidirectional. Disrupted sleep-wake cycles in the host will cause disturbances in the patterns of the circadian rhythm of the microbiome. Conversely, disruptions of the microbiome clock can lead to sleep-wake disturbances. The clock genes of the microbiome are not influenced by light but rather by cell metabolism. If the there is a continuous supply of food for the bacteria, their daily cycle becomes disrupted, including changes in the microbial population balance. This favors conditions that lead to chronic inflammation in the intestines. As we have seen, chronic inflammation is implicated in a great number of diseases. When gut bacteria have regular but limited access to food, they are able to synchronize their metabolic activities in a normal fashion. Yet another reason to adhere to age-old, time-tested, daily rhythms.

It is fascinating to realize that millennia ago, the Chinese realized that each organ in the body had its own time frame of peak functioning. This is

---

33. Yuanyuan Li, Yanli Hao, Fang Fan, and Bin Zhang, "The Role of Microbiome in Insomnia, Circadian Disturbance. and Depression," *Frontiers in Psychiatry* 9 (2018): 669, https://doi.org/10.3389/fpsyt.2018.00669.

known as the twenty-four-hour clock and describes the way in which the body's qi cycles through all the organ systems in the same sequence every day. Science has shown us that the ancient concept of naturally repeating body rhythms is correct. In keeping with the philosophy of the Dao, living in harmony with our body clocks is essential to optimal health.

Common Digestive and Metabolic Illnesses

In this section, we will be defining and describing the most common digestive diseases as well as the metabolic illnesses, diabetes, and obesity. In the following chapters we will address the integrative management of these conditions. There are a great many more digestive and metabolic diseases that we could discuss, but we cannot possibly cover them all in sufficient depth. We have specifically excluded gastrointestinal cancers, but we would like to remind you that all persistent GI symptoms, as well as unexplained weight loss, fever, and night sweats require evaluation by a Western medical professional. We have chosen to limit our discussion to those digestive and metabolic conditions that take a huge toll on large segments of our society and for which we feel the integration of Eastern and Western medicine will make the greatest positive impact.

Digestive Illnesses

The chronic digestive illnesses that affect the greatest number of Americans are:[34]
- Peptic (stomach) ulcer disease (fifteen million people)
- Irritable bowel syndrome (fifteen million people)
- Gastroesophageal reflux disease (GERD) (sixty million people)
- Chronic constipation (sixty-three million people)

Other gastrointestinal illness such as Crohn's disease, ulcerative colitis, and diverticular disease are less common, but can be equally painful and even more serious conditions.

---

34. National Institute of Diabetes and Digestive and Kidney Diseases, "Digestive Diseases Statistics for the United States," https://www.niddk.nih.gov/health-information/health-statistics/digestive-diseases, accessed August 16, 2017 and January 1, 2020.

There is another type of chronic digestive illness that people commonly experience—indigestion. This is also known as dyspepsia. Indigestion is really more of a symptom than a diagnosis. It is the word that people use to describe a GI condition in which they experience a variety of uncomfortable sensations. Nearly everyone has had indigestion at one time or another. It's a feeling of discomfort or a burning feeling in your upper abdomen. You may have slight stomach pain, belching, or bloating. You may feel that the food in your stomach takes a long time to go down. Your stomach may feel distended. You may also feel nauseated or even throw up.

Some people may get indigestion from eating too much food too fast, or eating high-fat foods. Indigestion can also occur if you eat when you are stressed. Smoking or drinking too much alcohol can also cause indigestion. Some medication can cause indigestion (this information can be found on the medication information sheet that comes with your medication). If you feel tired, are dehydrated, have ongoing stress, or have food sensitivities, you may be prone to indigestion. Any problem in the digestive tract and abdomen can lead to symptoms of indigestion. This is why the term is a better descriptor than it is a diagnosis.

At the end of the last century, Western medicine started to group these dyspeptic symptoms into subtypes based on their patterns.[35] These subtypes are known as ulcer-like, reflux-like, and dysmotility-like. The ulcer-like subtype encompasses conditions that feature abdominal pain. Reflux-like subtypes demonstrate symptoms of burning or having food come back up into the esophagus, possibly resulting in chest pain. Dysmotility-like subtypes present with bowel transit times that are either too fast or too slow, resulting in either diarrhea or constipation. These are generalities and it is important to remember that these classifications are descriptive and there is a lot of overlap. Still, these distinctions help clinicians formulate a plan for investigation, diagnosis, and treatment.

Sometimes, there is difficulty arriving at a diagnosis. This is extremely frustrating for the patient and physician alike. The patient is clearly having symptoms, but there are no findings to support a known diagnosis in

---

35. S. L. Grainger, H. J. Klass, M.O. Rake, and J. G. Williams, "Prevalence of Dyspepsia: The Epidemiology of Overlapping Symptoms," *Postgraduate Medical Journal* 70, no. 821 (Mar. 1994): 154–161, https://doi.org/10.1136/pgmj.70.821.154.

Western medicine. All the blood work and imaging are normal. Even when the patient undergoes a procedure where the GI specialist can see the lining of the gut, no abnormalities are found. In decades past, many patients were told that their symptoms were "all in their head." We now realize that conditions that have no obvious structural etiology are, in fact, related to a dysfunction of the organ system. The gut is simply not working properly. This is called a functional disorder and there are many, many reasons for this to occur. Some functional illnesses are caused by food choices that are not compatible with your digestive system and cause an imbalance in the microbiome. Others can be caused by stress, overwork, disrupted sleep, and past emotional trauma. All these disturbances can change the way the enteric nervous system works and how the gut functions.

Factors that Influence Intestinal Function and Motility

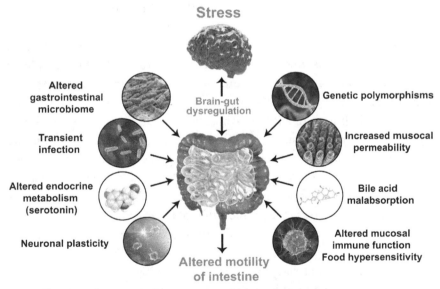

Illustration by Katerynakon, courtesy of Dreamstime.

Think of functional disorders in any organ system like your car's "check engine" light. Something is wrong and you need to pay attention to your body, mind, and spirit in order to get to the root of the problem. Eastern medicine is ideal for treating functional disorders. It uses acupuncture, meditation, qigong, and taiji to restore balance to the organs, as well as the enteric and central nervous system. Western medicine has discovered that often the root of the problem is chronic inflammation. Your gut is particularly susceptible to inflammation since its lining is the interface between trillions of microbes and the interior of your body.

When all is functioning normally, the bacteria and other organisms in your intestines do not present a problem. There is a mechanism in place whereby specialized immune cells called dendritic cells monitor the population of bacteria in your gut. The dendritic cells are able to do this because they are located immediately beneath the inner lining of your intestines and extend long "tentacles" through an intricate mucus bilayer into the interior of the gut. These "tentacles" have receptors that act as sensors and are part of the communication system between your microbiome and your immune system. It is as though the dendritic cells are sampling the microbiome, like officials taking a census. When the dendritic cells sense an infiltration of dangerous bacteria, they notify the immune system to mount an inflammatory response to keep the intruders at bay.[36]

The mucus bilayer protects the lining of the intestine. The bilayer is composed of a thick inner layer that acts as a barrier and a thin outer layer that houses the majority of your microbiome. This arrangement keeps the microbes from triggering the immune system of the gut directly. When microbes do breach this inner layer, certain molecules of their cell wall interact with your immune cells. Through this interaction, your immune system will judge how intensely it should respond to the intrusion. Lipopolysaccharides (LPS) are just one of these cell-wall molecules and are found on pathogenic gram-negative bacteria. They are important because they are able to increase the permeability of the gut and allow an influx of microbes that will interact with the immune system, leading to an increase in inflammation.[37]

It has been found that people who eat a diet high in animal fat tend to have more gram-negative bacteria in their intestines. Also, those who eat minimal plant-based fiber lack a certain bacteria (*Akkermansia muciniphilia*) that would normally increase the thickness and improve the quality of the inner mucus layer. This combination of dietary habits is like a

---

36. Mayer, 98.
37. Mayer, 98.

Increased Intestinal Permeability

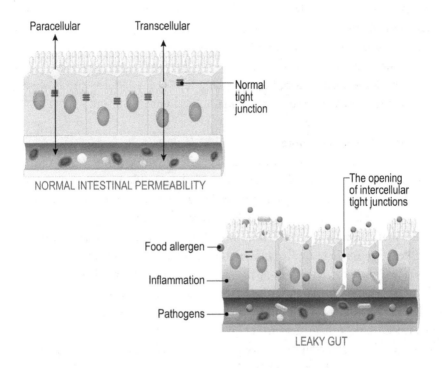

Illustration by Designua, courtesy of Dreamstime.

one-two punch, rendering the interface between you and your microbiome vulnerable to breaches in both mucus layer and gut lining. As the gut gets more permeable, incoming microbes or their signaling molecules trigger the intestine's immune system, which produces inflammatory cytokines. Cytokines promote acute inflammation in the gut, but can also promote inflammation in the brain, either by activating the vagus nerve or by traveling through the bloodstream directly to the brain. Here they can cause more inflammation and promote neurodegenerative diseases such as Alzheimer's and Parkinson's disease.[38]

---

38. Mayer, 100.

This inflammatory process has been implicated in many conditions that involve an exaggerated immune response. The theory is that the immune system that was triggered by foreign microbial molecules then starts to mistakenly attack human tissue. This may be the basis of autoimmune diseases such as inflammatory bowel disease, celiac disease, lupus, Hashimoto's thyroiditis, type-1 diabetes, and multiple sclerosis, to name but a few.

Now that we have discussed GI tract disease in general terms, let's describe some specific conditions. In chapter 3 we will delve into how you can integrate Eastern and Western medicine to heal your gut.

Irritable Bowel Syndrome
Irritable bowel syndrome (IBS), which is not the same thing as inflammatory bowel disease (IBD), is a condition that is typified by bowel changes such as diarrhea or constipation as well as abdominal pain. This is a functional disorder. After a full investigation by your doctor, there will be no abnormal findings on lab testing, imaging, or direct visualization of the inside of your GI tract. This is in stark contrast to inflammatory bowel disease (IBD) where there is clear evidence of damage and disease.

For whatever reason, with IBS, the brain-gut communication is disrupted, causing the bowel to be more sensitive and leading to pain and bloating. A significant feature of IBS is that bowel motility is either too fast, too slow, or alternating between the two. If your bowel peristalsis is too fast, you are said to have IBS with diarrhea (IBS-D) and if it is too slow, you have IBS with constipation (IBS-C). If you have a combination, the name for this condition is IBS with mixed bowel habits (IBS-M). There are specific criteria for these diagnoses that describe what percentage of your bowel movements are either too loose or too hard on a day when you have abnormal stools. Many people have normal bowel movements and only have problems some of the time.

There is no obvious reason why IBS occurs. It can start following a bacterial or parasitic infection of the intestines or if there is an imbalance in the bacteria of your small intestine (small intestinal bacterial overgrowth, known as SIBO). Food sensitivities can play a role. A common feature is a history of traumatic early life experiences such as physical or sexual abuse. There may also be a history of psychoemotional problems and other pain syndromes such as fibromyalgia and chronic fatigue syndrome.

While IBS can occur at any age, it often begins when people are in their teens or reach early adulthood. Women are affected more often than men. The good news is that IBS is treatable with integrative medicine using various Eastern and Western methods to reduce stress and synchronize the enteric and central nervous system.

Celiac Disease

Celiac disease is a condition caused by damage to the lining of the small intestine. This damage comes from a reaction to eating gluten, a plant protein found in wheat and some other grains like rye and barley. It is also found in food made from these ingredients.

Celiac Disease

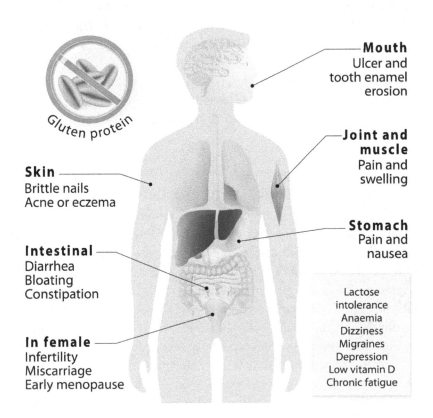

Gluten protein

Mouth
Ulcer and
tooth enamel
erosion

**Joint and
muscle**
Pain and
swelling

Skin
Brittle nails
Acne or eczema

Stomach
Pain and
nausea

Intestinal
Diarrhea
Bloating
Constipation

Lactose
intolerance
Anaemia
Dizziness
Migraines
Depression
Low vitamin D
Chronic fatigue

In female
Infertility
Miscarriage
Early menopause

Illustration by Designua, courtesy of Dreamstime.

Celiac disease is an immune system disorder, but it is not an allergy. When people with celiac disease eat foods with gluten, their immune system reacts by damaging the villi, the part of intestinal wall that absorb nutrients. This may cause a number of symptoms such as bloating, abdominal swelling and pain, constipation, chronic diarrhea, excessive gas, nausea, vomiting, and fatty stools. Some symptoms may not even involve the gut. These include an itchy and blistering skin rash, headaches, infertility, recurrent miscarriage, mouth sores, seizures, fatigue, and joint pain. People with celiac disease may have other immune disorders such as Hashimoto's thyroiditis leading to hypothyroidism, type-1 diabetes, and Addison's disease, which affects the adrenals.

About 1 in 141 people have celiac disease, but its exact cause is not well defined. We know that it happens in people who carry certain genes that are quite common and present in about one-third of the population. We also know that these people need to be eating gluten to manifest the disease. What we don't know is why some people are severely affected and others are not, aside from how much gluten they eat. It seems that being breastfed for longer confers some protection in that the symptoms appear later in life. The age at which you started eating gluten also has some bearing. There may be environmental triggers that influence the severity of the disease.

Gastroesophageal Reflux Disease

Gastroesophageal reflux disease (GERD) is a condition in which the chyme in your stomach backs up into your esophagus, causing a burning sensation when the stomach acid comes into contact with the esophageal lining. This is commonly known as heartburn or acid indigestion. Everyone experiences this once in a while, often after a heavy meal with foods that loosen the esophageal sphincter. Such foods include chocolate, alcohol, and even something as seemingly benign as mint tea. Certain medications have this effect, like antidepressants, sedatives, analgesics, asthma medications, and blood pressure medications.

People who are more likely to have chronic problems with GERD are those who are overweight or smoke. Those who have a hiatal hernia can also experience heartburn. In this condition, the upper part of the stomach moves above the diaphragm into the chest cavity.

Symptoms of GERD include chest pain or abdominal pain, nausea, trouble swallowing, vomiting, bad breath, and problems breathing. Sometimes people who suffer from GERD dismiss their symptoms as simply heartburn, but occasionally these symptoms can be associated with serious heart and lung conditions. If your symptoms persist or are complicated by vomiting of blood, be sure to seek medical attention.

Crohn's Disease

Crohn's disease is an illness that results from inflammation of the digestive tract, most commonly from the ileum at the end of the small intestine to the cecum at the beginning of the colon. Although it certainly can be found in parts of the GI tract from the mouth to the anus, this is less common. The areas of the gut damaged by this condition are found in patches. In contrast, the damage caused by inflammation in the colon found with ulcerative colitis is seen in a long, continuous tract. Both Crohn's disease and ulcerative colitis are types of inflammatory bowel disease (IBD). It is worth noting that IBD is a structural disease with specific abnormalities discovered during the evaluation of the condition, whereas in irritable bowel syndrome (IBS) the problem arises in the way the bowel functions, not its structure.

Symptoms of Crohn's disease can vary between mild to severe. They tend to flare up, and then wane. The symptoms and signs include crampy abdominal pain, diarrhea, blood in the stool, fever, weight loss. Because Crohn's disease is a type of autoimmune condition, there can be other areas in the body that show signs of inflammation along with the bowel. These include the eyes, skin, and joints.

The exact cause of Crohn's disease is not known, though there are many factors that seem to be involved. These include a genetic pre-disposition toward the condition as seen in Caucasians and people of Eastern European Jewish descent, immune system dysregulation, and environmental triggers such as smoking. Where you live may also play a role, as people who live in urban and industrialized areas are more likely to have Crohn's than those who live in rural areas. Most people with Crohn's disease are diagnosed around the age of thirty.

Ulcerative Colitis

Just as the name implies, ulcerative colitis is a disease in which inflammatory ulcers affect the lining of the colon. Like Crohn's disease, it is a subtype of inflammatory bowel disease (IBD), but it is only found in the colon and rectum. The lesions of ulcerative colitis tend to be contiguous rather than patchy. Over time, it could involve the entire large intestine.

Symptoms of ulcerative colitis can range in severity, depending upon the amount of inflammation present. Signs and symptoms can include diarrhea (with or without blood and pus), abdominal discomfort ranging from cramping to intense pain, rectal pain (with or without bloody stools), tenesmus (inability to pass stool, even if you feel urgency to do so), sudden need to pass stool, weight loss, fever, and fatigue. Complications associated with ulcerative colitis can include rectal bleeding that is bad enough to require transfusion, dehydration, ulcers that go through the whole thickness of the colon and create a hole (perforation), and increased risk of colon cancer. As with Crohn's disease, this inflammatory process can affect your skin, eyes, and joints.

No one knows precisely what causes ulcerative colitis, but poor diet and stress can exacerbate the condition. This inflammatory disease may start through a misinterpretation by your immune system. What may begin as a reasonable attempt by the immune system to fight an infecting microbe can go awry if the cells that line the colon are targeted by accident. This is a common theory linking all autoimmune diseases. You may be at risk for ulcerative colitis if anyone in your family has this condition, if you are Caucasian, or are of Eastern European Jewish descent. Age at diagnosis varies widely from less than thirty years of age to over sixty.

Chronic Constipation

Every year, there are 2.5 million visits to primary care providers or specialists for the treatment of constipation. Everyone's bowel habits are slightly different, but if you have fewer than three stools per week that are hard, dry, and difficult to pass, you are probably constipated. Sometimes the stool looks like little rabbit pellets, and other times it may feel as though there is still more to come out.

Constipation is extremely common, especially in people who eat little or no fiber. Lack of physical activity also makes people more prone to constipation. Just a change in your usual daily routine can alter your bowel habits. Travel, especially if you become dehydrated along the way, can contribute to this, but is usually not a chronic problem.

Certain medications can cause constipation, and especially opioids, which slow down the movement of the bowels and increase the time it takes the stool to make it through the whole colon. During that time, more water is reabsorbed and the stools get drier. Other medications that increase the risk of constipation include any that contain calcium or aluminum, a type of blood pressure medication called a calcium channel blocker, iron supplements, and some antidepressants. Be sure to check the side effect list of any medication or supplement you are taking, especially if this condition arose after starting them.

You may also be prone to chronic constipation if you have an underlying health problem such as Parkinson's disease, diabetes, and hypothyroidism. Brain or spinal cord injuries can slow down bowel function. Some people are born with anatomical abnormalities that can lead to constipation.

Sometimes the problem is that the muscular sphincter of the rectum does not relax sufficiently. If you are continually in a situation where you cannot use the bathroom and end up holding your stools too long, you may lose the ability to sense when you need to defecate.

If you struggle with chronic constipation, you may have some rectal bleeding when you go to the bathroom. Usually that is from a hemorrhoid, a swollen area of veins at the anus, often caused by the increased pressure from straining to pass stool. It is important, though, to see your healthcare provider to make sure the blood is not coming from colon cancer. As we will see in chapter 3, a lot can be done to ease the discomfort of constipation from most causes, but first a tumor must be ruled out.

Diabetes Mellitus

Diabetes mellitus is a condition in which a person's sugar metabolism is impaired, leading to elevated sugar levels in the blood. The word "mellitus" means "sweet." As the blood sugar levels get higher, some of the sugar can be detected in the urine. In fact, before blood testing was available, doctors would taste the patient's urine. If it was sweet, the patient was diagnosed with diabetes mellitus. These days, it is more common to refer to this condition simply as diabetes.

Diabetes is associated with very serious complications, such as heart disease, stroke, blindness, kidney failure, and lower-limb amputation. This disease continues to increase at an alarming rate in the United States. In 2017, there were an estimated thirty million diabetics. By the time the CDC's National Diabetes Statistics Report for 2020 was released, that number had risen to thirty-four million. That means that roughly one in ten Americans are diabetic. Furthermore, eighty-eight million Americans are prediabetic, indicating that the way their bodies manage glucose is abnormal, but not to the point of being diagnosed as diabetic. Over 120 million of us have problems with glucose metabolism.[39] That's a ratio of one in three!

In 2012, the total estimated cost of diagnosed diabetes in the U.S. was $245 billion, but by 2017 the national cost was more than $327 billion. That represents an increase of about 33 percent in just five years. Average medical expenditures for people with diagnosed diabetes were about $16,750 per year. About $9,600 of this amount was attributed to diabetes. Average medical expenditures among people with diagnosed diabetes were about 2.3 times higher than expenditures for people without diabetes. In terms of healthcare dollars, $1 in every $7 is spent treating diabetes and its complications. Indirect costs from loss productivity are estimated to be as high as $90 billion.[40]

Diabetes can be classified into two main types, type 1 and type 2. Type-3 diabetes is the newer term that many scientists and doctors are ascribing to Alzheimer's disease. The molecular, biochemical, and cellular changes found in the brains of those affected by Alzheimer's can be attributed to the changes in sugar (glucose) metabolism found in diabetics.[41]

---

39. Centers for Disease Control, "National Diabetes Statistics Report for 2020," https://www.cdc.gov/diabetes/data/statistics/statistics-report.html, accessed March 18, 2020.

40. American Diabetes Association, "The Cost of Diabetes," https://www.diabetes.org/resources/statistics, accessed March 18, 2020.

41. Suzanne M. de la Monte, MD, MPH, and Jack R. Wands, "Alzheimer's Disease Is Type-3 Diabetes—Evidence Reviewed," *Journal of Diabetes Science and*

Type-1 diabetes accounts for approximately 10 percent of all diabetes in America with type-2 diabetes making up the remaining 90 percent. Type-3 diabetes would be considered in a different grouping because, while all people who have Alzheimer's disease would have evidence of impaired glucose metabolism in their brains, not all of these people would be diabetic.

With type-1 diabetes, the age of onset is usually younger (though this has changed in recent years as we will see). It comes on rapidly and is thought to have an immunologic or infectious cause. It is not necessarily associated with obesity and is always treated with insulin. In contrast, type-2 diabetes has a gradual onset and is commonly associated with obesity as well as a strong family predisposition toward the disease. It is one of the manifestations of oxidative stress and chronic inflammation that we discussed earlier.[42]

In type-1 diabetes the pancreas either does not make enough insulin or the insulin that is created is not structurally normal. Insulin is a vital hormone involved in the body's utilization of glucose (sugar). While the body also metabolizes other nutrients and molecules, glucose is arguably the most important. In fact, glucose is the main source of energy for the brain and is required for it to function normally. This is why when your blood sugar is low (a condition called hypoglycemia) you may experience headaches, dizziness, fatigue, or irritability. Some people may even become confused. Symptoms of this sort of diabetes include sudden increased urination, excessive thirst, weight loss, and fatigue. Without insulin, glucose cannot enter your cells and provide energy for normal body functioning. Until the identification of insulin by Canadian researchers Frederick Banting and Charles Best in 1921, patients with type-1 diabetes mellitus routinely died prematurely. Insulin is injected into the skin to allow the body to utilize the glucose that is derived from the food you eat. Type-1 diabetes is also known as insulin dependent diabetes mellitus (IDDM). While the inclusion of complementary lifestyle changes and East Asian therapies may decrease insulin

Technology 2, no. 6 (Nov. 2008): 1101–1113, https://doi.org/10.1177/193229680800200619, accessed April 9, 2017.

42. Richard Nahas, MD, "Type-2 Diabetes," in *Integrative Medicine*, 3rd ed., ed. David Rakel, MD, (Philadelphia: Saunders, Elsevier, 2012), 926.

requirements in type-1 diabetics, any adjustment in medications should be strictly prescribed by your physician.

In type-2 diabetes mellitus, known as non-insulin dependent diabetes mellitus (NIDDM), the pancreas does create insulin, but the cells are resistant to the insulin. In this situation, insulin cannot easily function mainly because a certain protein (GLUT-4) stays inside the cell rather than on the surface where it controls glucose transport. In patients with type-2 diabetes, insulin levels are actually high as the pancreas works harder producing more insulin in an effort to lower blood sugar levels to a normal range.

This sort of diabetes is seen most often in obese patients and is commonly treated with diet, exercise, and oral medications that make it easier for insulin to enter the cells or force the pancreas to make more insulin. But eventually, if corrective measures are insufficient or the patient is not compliant with lifestyle changes, the pancreas becomes exhausted and cannot keep up with the demand. This is why some patients who are type-2 diabetics are prescribed insulin as their disease process worsens.

Factors that increase your risk of developing insulin resistance and type-2 diabetes include obesity (especially if there is a lot fat around your abdomen), physical inactivity, eating too many refined carbohydrates, being diagnosed with diabetes during pregnancy, having a family history of diabetes, and smoking. Additionally, if you are of African, Latino, or Native American descent your genetics will predispose you to insulin resistance and type-2 diabetes. Some medications can elevate blood sugars and so, too, can some hormonal conditions. People with sleep problems, like sleep apnea, are also at risk.

Type-2 diabetes is often called adult-onset diabetes. Unfortunately, this has become something of a misnomer as more and more American children are being diagnosed with insulin-resistant diabetes. This increase in childhood diabetes has occurred because of the epidemic levels of obesity among the youth in this country. The incidence of childhood obesity has tripled in the past thirty years.[43] Obesity is strongly correlated with the onset of type-2 diabetes. According to the American Diabetes Association 2011 National Diabetes Fact Sheet, about one in every four hundred

---

43. Center for Disease Control and Prevention, "Healthy Youth," https://www.cdc.gov/healthyschools/obesity/index.html, accessed March 18, 2020.

children and adolescents currently has diabetes. Additionally, it is estimated that one in three children born in the year 2000 will develop type-2 diabetes in their lifetime (nearly one in two for ethnic minorities).[44] As we have already discussed, one in three Americans already have problems metabolizing glucose when you consider those who have prediabetes along with the diabetics. If you are prediabetic, you can cut your risk of becoming diabetic in half by maintaining a healthy weight and engaging in regular physical activity. In the coming chapters, we will show you how.

Whether you have prediabetes or either type of diabetes mellitus, you should use all available resources to normalize your glucose metabolism to avoid serious and potentially life-threatening complications. Here are a few sobering statistics:[45]

If you have diabetes, compared to someone who does not:
- You are twice as likely to have a heart attack.
- You are twice as likely to have stroke.
- You are more likely to have high blood pressure.
- You have a one-in-four chance of having eye problems that could lead to blindness.
- You are more likely to develop kidney failure, which can require dialysis or transplant.
- You are more likely to need your foot or lower leg amputated due to poor wound healing and subsequent gangrene.
- You have a higher risk of developing Alzheimer's disease or other dementias. In fact, as mentioned at the beginning of this section, there is such a strong similarity in the biochemical changes that occur in the progression of type-2 diabetes and Alzheimer's disease, that some researchers consider Alzheimer's disease to be diabetes of the brain, often called type-3 diabetes.[46]

---

44. K. M. Venkat Narayan, et al, "Lifetime Risk for Diabetes Mellitus in the United States," *Journal of the American Medical Association* 290 (2003): 1884–1890.

45. American Diabetes Association, "Statistics about Diabetes," http://www.diabetes.org/diabetes-basics/statistics/, accessed Aug 11, 2016.

46. F. G. de Felice and S. T. Ferreira, "Inflammation, Defective Insulin Signaling, and Mitochondrial Dysfunction as Common Molecular Denominators Connecting

These is a very scary list of potential complications but the diagnosis of prediabetes or diabetes is a golden opportunity for you to take charge of your health. While even type-1 diabetics can improve their health and quality of life, those of you who suffer from variants of type-2 diabetes have the greatest chance to be free of medications and the ravages of this disease.

You *can* avoid the serious complications of diabetes. There are many strategies that you can implement from both a Western and Eastern perspective. We will discuss these approaches in chapter 4. Please keep in mind that it is imperative to continue your insulin or oral medications at the prescribed dose unless your physician tells you otherwise. You will find that as you put the following suggestions into practice, your blood

---

Type-2 Diabetes to Alzheimer Disease," *Diabetes* 63, no. 7 (Jul. 2014): 2262–2272, http://dx.doi.org/10.2337/db13-1954, accessed Aug 11, 2016.

Types of Diabetes

Type I diabetes

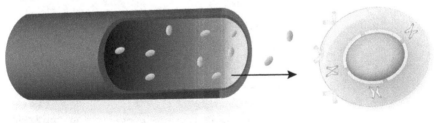

Type II diabetes

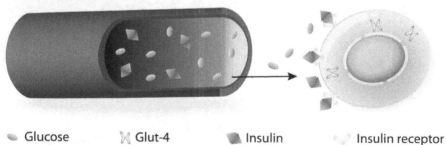

Glucose   Glut-4   Insulin   Insulin receptor

Illustration by Designua, courtesy of Dreamstime.

sugars will be better controlled. Your sugars may even end up being on the low side. If this occurs, call your doctor to ask for guidance in adjusting your medication dosage. You may find yourself needing less and less medication through the integration of Western and Eastern medicine.

Obesity

Rates of obesity in the United States continue to rise, in spite of the clearly documented risks to our health and well-being. As of 2000, approximately 30 percent of Americans were obese as measured by body mass index (BMI). By 2010, that percentage had increased to 35 percent and by 2015 it had reached 40 percent.[47] If you look at the rate of increase, you will notice that in the five years between 2010 and 2015 the obesity rate increased as much as it had in the ten years prior. The acceleration of the prevalence of this condition is nothing short of alarming.

When you take into account all the dangerous conditions that are associated with obesity, such as heart disease and diabetes, it is no wonder that obesity is considered the second leading cause of preventable death in Western societies.

In the past few years, obesity has been classified as a disease. Some would say that obesity is actually a symptom of metabolic dysregulation. Whichever side of the argument you are on, one thing is clear. Obesity, particularly abdominal obesity, is associated with many chronic life-threatening diseases, more admissions to the hospital, higher prescription costs, and poor quality of life.

Every year more than 300,000 Americans die as a consequence of obesity-related illnesses or complications. Any physician will tell you that being obese can make your medical care more problematic. Not only are the risks of having a heart attack, stroke, or diabetes higher for the obese patient, the chances that something will go wrong during treatment are also increased. This particularly applies to procedures, surgeries, and even childbirth.

The bottom-line cause of the obesity epidemic is far from clear. A 2016 study looked at dietary data from over 36,000 adults and the physical

---

47. Craig M. Hales, MD, et al. "Prevalence of Obesity among Adults and Youth: United States, 2015–2016," NCHS Data Brief No. 288, October 2017, https://www.cdc.gov/nchs/data/databriefs/db288.pdf.

activity data from over 14,000 adults, covering the years from 1971 to 2008 and 1988 to 2006, respectively. Some very interesting observations were made. In essence, comparing groups of similar individuals, the 2006 cohort were about 10 percent heavier than their counterparts from 1988, even though the caloric intake, macronutrient ratio (protein, fat, and carbohydrate), and physical activity were comparable.[48]

Clearly, there is more to weight gain than simply taking in more energy than you use. Obesity is considered a multifactorial condition that is influenced by genetics, dietary intake, levels of physical activity, environmental metabolic disruptors, altered gastrointestinal function, chronic inflammation, behavior, and disequilibrium of the human microbiome. Our understanding of why people gain excessive amounts of weight is continuing to evolve. One thing *is* becoming increasingly obvious: losing weight and maintaining a healthy body mass index is not simply a matter of willpower.

A considerable amount of research has been done to determine what controls appetite and what makes a person want to eat. More importantly, scientists have been investigating what makes a person *stop* eating. The "starting" and "stopping" mechanisms are the "appetite" and "satiety" control centers of the brain. These centers are mostly located in the area of the brain called the hypothalamus. The hypothalamus communicates with the rest of the body and helps orchestrate the intake, digestion, and utilization of food. The brain is not the only organ involved in regulating energy intake and metabolism. It is now known that fat cells have input, too.

At one time, adipose cells were thought to be simply a storage site for excess calories. Actually, fat is metabolically active and now considered to be the body's largest hormone-producing organ. Hormones produced by adipose tissue are called adipokines. One adipokine called adiponectin has anti-inflammatory effects, but the more fat a person carries, the lower the levels of adiponectin. This loss of the protective effect of adiponectin leads to a state of chronic inflammation. It is thought that this is the common pathway for the development of other diseases such as diabetes,

48. Ruth E. Brown, et al. "Secular Differences in the Association between Caloric Intake, Macronutrient Intake, and Physical Activity with Obesity," *Obesity Research and Clinical Practice* 10, no. 3 (May–June 2016): 241–255, https://doi.org/10.1016/jorcp.2015.08.007.

hypertension, and heart disease. In some respects, it is difficult to know which came first, obesity or inflammation; however, there is evidence that overeating may be the culprit.

Sensing when to eat and when to stop is also a complicated process. The hormone pair that controls appetite and satiety is ghrelin and leptin. Ghrelin is a hormone that increases appetite. It is secreted before meals and decreases after meals. Leptin is made within the fat cells (adipose tissue) and released into the blood stream. When adipose tissue increases, so do leptin levels in the blood. This tells the hypothalamus to send neural signals to decrease food intake and increase energy metabolism until a normal balance is restored. Conversely, when adipose tissue has decreased below what the body considers to be its norm, leptin levels will decrease, food intake will increase, and energy metabolism will decrease until the body once again has achieved equilibrium.

Normally, this balance is well maintained, with leptin and ghrelin levels moving in opposite directions like a see-saw, but with obesity these hormonal signals have gone awry. People who are obese often have high levels of leptin and low levels of ghrelin. When someone is obese, there are enough calories being taken in and enough stored fat to ensure that the body will have energy to survive. The subsequent high leptin levels in the body should be a signal to decrease the amount of food eaten and increase energy metabolism. The problem is that, in obese people, the cells in the hypothalamus that would normally set these changes in motion have become resistant to leptin. No matter how high the leptin levels are, the brain is not receiving the correct information. The brain is not receiving the signal that normally tells it that a person has eaten and is full. Therefore, that person never really feels full. The leptin levels remain high and therefore the ghrelin levels stay low.

Above and beyond leptin resistance, there are many reasons why people overeat. Researchers point out that there are many factors at work, including the endocannabinoid system, the reward system in the brain, and the disruptive influence of chronic inflammation.[49] While hormonal imbalances

---

49. Martin G. Myers, Jr., Rudolph L. Leibel, Randy J. Seeley, and Michael W. Schwartz, "Obesity and Leptin Resistance: Distinguishing Cause from Effect", *Trends in Endocrinology and Metabolism*, 2010 Nov; 21(11): 643-651. Doi: 10.1016/j.rem.2010.08.002.

have been found in obese people, sometimes the problem is not strictly related to hormonal biochemistry. Chronic sleep deprivation has been associated with cravings for simple carbohydrates and excessive eating. Many people overeat when they are under stress or are emotionally upset.

Medications can also play a role in promoting obesity. There are many prescription drugs with side effect profiles that include weight gain through a variety of different mechanisms. The medication may increase your appetite by altering your brain's perception of fullness after you eat. You may be eating the way you always have, but you do not feel like you have eaten enough. The medication may change the way your body processes fluids and make you retain water, or it may increase fat storage or slow down your metabolism. Many medications cause fatigue or weakness, simply making you less active so you burn fewer calories. If you have gained weight after starting a new medication or are struggling to lose weight while taking drugs that are known to cause weight gain, your physician can find suitable alternatives.

Some medications that list weight gain as a known side effect are listed below.

Heart/Blood Pressure Medications:
- acebutolol (Sectral)
- atenolol (Tenormin)
- metoprolol (Lopressor, Toprol XL)
- propranolol (Inderal)

Diabetes Medications:
- glimepiride (Amaryl)
- glipizide (Glucotrol)
- glyburide (Diabeta, Micronase)
- insulin
- nateglinide (Starlix)
- pioglitazone (Actos)
- replaglinide (Prandin)

Migraine Medications:
- amitriptyline (Elavil)
- nortriptyline (Aventyl, Pamelor)

Anti-Seizure Medications:

- valproic acid (Depacon, Depakote, Stavzor)
- pregabalin (Lyrica)—also used to treat pain syndromes

Corticosteroids:
- methylprednisolone (Medrol)
- prednisolone (Orapred, Pediapred, Prelone)
- prednisone (Deltasone, Prednicot, Sterapred)

Antidepressant Medications:
- citalopram (Celexa)
- fluoxetine (Prozac)
- fluvoxamine (Luvox)
- mirtazapine (Remeron)
- paroxetine (Paxil)
- sertraline (Zoloft)

Mood Stabilizing Medications:
- clozapine (Clozaril)
- lithium (Eskalith, Lithobid)
- olanzapine (Zyprexa)
- quetiapine (Seroquel)
- resperidone (Risperdal)

Birth Control:
- medroxyprogesterone (Depoprovera)

And then there is the microbiome. Recall that your specific microbiome may be better than others at extracting calories from food. That 10-to-15-percent increase in calorie absorption is enough to tip the balance from health to disease. Also, if your microbiome is not making enough short chain fatty acids, your metabolism may not be running optimally, and you may have more cravings for calorie dense foods. As we have also discussed, your microbiome is intricately in tune with your sleep-wake cycles and, if disturbed, can disrupt your sleep and contribute to weight gain through suboptimal metabolic processes.

To top it all off, gaining weight changes your body chemistry and physiology so that you are more likely to gain more weight. Being sleep deprived can lead to weight gain, and being overweight will disrupt your sleep, leading to further weight gain. Being obese can cause significant emotional upset, resulting in the release of stress hormones that increase appetite and promote the storage of calories as fat.

As you can see, obesity is complicated. But, however complex the cause of the problem, there is a solution. No matter how high your starting point, you can become healthier. Even a reduction of 5 to 10 percent of your total weight can decrease your risk of chronic disease. Use the Eastern and Western recommendations in chapter 5 to help tackle your weight problem and increase your quality of life.

CHAPTER **3**

The True Wellness Approach to Gastrointestinal Problems

T HE MOST FRUSTRATING PART about gastrointestinal problems is that often there are no abnormal findings. Your lab tests are normal. Your ultrasounds or CT scans are normal. Even when your doctor can see the lining of your gut by performing a special procedure called an endoscopy, the inner wall your intestines are normal. On paper, you look perfect, but you are still having symptoms. Now what?

A lot of patients come to us asking this question. Although we will discuss specific treatments for specific conditions, this chapter is primarily for those of you who are still struggling with GI disorders that defy diagnosis or have not improved with conventional care. Of course, everyone can benefit from the step-by-step strategies we are about to describe because this is a whole-systems approach to healing.

First, the following advice assumes that you have already seen your healthcare provider. Your visit should have included a thorough interview about your symptoms, including any changes in your bowel habits, with questions regarding level of pain, blood in your vomit or stool, and any travel history. A physical examination should have been performed. If any tests were ordered, you should have received those results and an explanation of their meaning. These tests could include blood work, stool samples, x-rays, ultrasounds, or CT scans at your provider's discretion. You may even have already undergone an upper or lower endoscopy to visualize inside of your stomach and intestines. If so, your doctor will have told you what was seen.

At this point, hopefully a diagnosis was reached and you are improving by following your doctor's advice. Even if this is the case, keep reading. The integration of Eastern and Western modalities can speed your recovery and prevent relapses. Unfortunately, you may be among the many patients who still feel unwell, despite excellent conventional care, or whose diagnosis remains unknown. For you, this chapter is particularly important.

Digestive illness can be very tricky to sort out. Sometimes people are unable to pinpoint the exact cause of their symptoms. Is it the food you are eating? Is it chronic stress at work or at home? Is your microbiome out of balance? Are you sleeping enough? Are you a shift worker? Are your symptoms a side effect of your medications? Each of these questions must be honestly answered for you to find a solution.

In the next section we will outline a dietary method that can help you determine whether there is a particular food or food group that is the root of your troubles. It will take weeks to work through this approach. In the meantime, we recommend that you read and implement the suggestions outlined in the remainder of this chapter, using these techniques simultaneously. One might argue that it is more scientific to try each approach sequentially to understand the cause of the problem and the most effective solution. This is certainly a valid viewpoint; however, it is our opinion that the goal is to alleviate suffering as quickly as possible. These methods will work together, synergistically, to accelerate your healing.

The Four-Phase Elimination Diet

Almost anyone can do an elimination diet, but children, pregnant women, and people with eating disorders like anorexia should not. An elimination diet is not a weight loss diet. It is a diagnostic tool that you can use to determine the foods that are most healing for your body. You may have heard of an elimination diet before. This is a method of dietary detective work. Think of your illness as a mystery that needs to be solved. You must be patient and observant. Did Sherlock Holmes rush through a case? Never. He paid careful attention to the smallest detail and he took as much time as he needed to solve the mystery. If you are organized and attentive, you can find the clues you need to heal.

Phase 1—Preparation

Just as the name implies, an elimination diet focuses on eliminating foods from your diet that may be causing your symptoms. There are several ways to go about this. First, you need to know exactly what you are already eating by keeping a food diary. We will give you a food diary template later in this chapter or you may want to create your own spreadsheet. It is useful to spend a couple of weeks simply documenting everything you eat and drink on a daily basis and noting any symptoms you may have. As odd as this may sound, include a description of your stools. The main thing to remember is that the symptoms you experience may not be due to the food you ate that same day. It could have been something you ingested up to seventy-two hours prior. You can see why digestive problems related to food intolerances are sometimes so difficult to sort out.

You may or may not see a pattern emerge during these first two weeks, but you will have a clear idea about the quality of your diet. Are you eating a lot of processed foods with chemical additives? How many fruits and vegetables do you eat every day? Are your meals heavy on dairy and animal proteins? How much water do you drink? Which foods would be the most difficult for you to give up? Make note of the foods you crave or use to comfort yourself, as these may be the very foods that are causing your symptoms.

If you are honest, you will see where you can make changes that will benefit your gut. Sometimes simply eating more plants and less of everything else is enough to get your symptoms under control. A study done in Britain found that 70 percent of people with food intolerances improved their symptoms just by eating healthy foods for two weeks. This improvement occurred without completely eliminating anything. The study subjects were merely asked to reduce their intake of soda, processed foods, and caffeine, as well as increase their intake of whole grains, vegetables, and fruits.[1]

---

1. Suhani Bora, MD, and J. Adam Rindfleisch, MPhil, "The Elimination Diet," in *Integrative Medicine*, 4th ed., ed. David Rakel (Philadelpha: Elsevier, 2018), 853.

Phase 2—Enhancement

For the next two weeks in Phase 2, enhance your diet. Commit to eating more foods that nourish your GI tract and your microbiome and less of the foods that have been shown to be detrimental. One way to immediately decrease your intake of processed food is to cook at home using simple ingredients. You have more control over what you are putting in your body.

Drink less soda and caffeinated beverages. Increase your plant and whole grain consumption. One easy way to do this is by filling half your plate with non-starchy vegetables and one quarter of your plate with starchy vegetables or whole grains, leaving the last quarter for some protein of your choice.

Continue to diligently record the foods you eat and drink, along with any symptoms that may occur and the appearance of your stool. After two weeks, you may notice a decrease in the severity and frequency of symptoms and a normalization of your bowel habits. If your problems go away entirely, these are all the dietary changes you may need to make! If you are still having troublesome symptoms, move on to Phase 3.

Phase 3—Elimination

This phase is where you need to tap into your inner Sherlock Holmes. There are three ways you can approach this. You can eliminate one food or food group, multiple food groups at once, or eat only a limited list of foods that are very unlikely to cause symptoms. There are benefits and disadvantages of each approach. Here are some considerations to help you decide which method to use.

Eliminate One Food or Food Group. This method is the least restrictive and the best place to start if you already suspect that one food is the main culprit causing your symptoms. While continuing your new healthy way of eating, simply avoid that one food and document how you feel over several days. If you have no inkling where to start, you could eliminate a food group that commonly causes GI symptoms, such as dairy or gluten. The main advantage of this approach is that it is easiest to stick with and be consistent. The disadvantage is that it may take a while to test foods one by one in this manner. That would be particularly troubling if your symptoms are moderate to severe and not improving. If this were the case, a more restrictive approach would be better. If your condition has improved, move on to Phase 4. If there is no change, you need to eliminate more foods simultaneously as described next.

Eliminate Multiple Food Groups. This approach is significantly more restrictive. The idea is that you are trying to avoid as many inflammation-causing foods as possible, all at the same time. Such foods include:

- corn
- dairy
- gluten (a protein found in wheat, barley, rye, spelt, and kamut)
- eggs
- peanuts
- shellfish
- alcohol
- coffee

Eliminate these foods for two weeks and continue with your enhanced food plan. Continue to log your food intake, symptoms, and bowel habits.

If your condition improves considerably, move on to Phase 4. If there is no change or insufficient change in your symptoms, try removing certain foods that tend to cause bloating and gas. These are foods that contain particular types of carbohydrates and sugars that are not well absorbed when the gut lining is inflamed. They can consequently cause abdominal pain and distention. As a group, these foods are known as FODMAPs. This is an acronym for **F**ermentable **O**ligo-, **D**i-, and **M**onosaccharides **a**nd **P**olyols. The oligo-, di-, and monosaccharides are all short-chain carbohydrates, meaning they have less than four carbon atoms. The bacteria in your gut easily ferment these short-chain fatty acids and polyols, but the hydrogen atoms that are subsequently produced can cause bloating, pain, and gas.

Some short-chain carbohydrates are lactose, fructose, fructans, and galactans. Trying to eliminate all foods containing these molecules as well as foods that contain polyols would make for a very onerous and restrictive food regimen. Most people would give it up completely. Some people might even become malnourished if they stuck with it long term. This is because almost all foods that contain FODMAPs are highly nutritious!

Here are a few examples of FODMAPs based on the short-carbohydrate or polyol that predominates:

Lactose: dairy products
Fructose: apples, pears, peaches, fruit juices, honey
Fructans: wheat, rye, asparagus, broccoli, garlic, onions, lettuce, beetroot, artichokes, brussels sprouts, cabbage
Galactans: chickpeas, lentils, soy products
Polyols: apples, cherries, pears, watermelon, cauliflower, snow peas, sweeteners ending in –ol such as mannitol, xylitol, sorbitol

It is inadvisable to eliminate all these foods. Experienced gastroenterologists, such as Dr. Gerard Mullin at Johns Hopkins, recommend you start by avoiding the FODMAPs that give the majority of patients the most problems. These are wheat, apples, pears, and raw onions. He also suggests that for the other foods that you eat small portions until you are sure your gut can handle more. Do not eat a large number of FODMAPs at one time. Regarding fruit, it should be ripe. Cooked foods are more easily digested than raw foods.[2]

Selectively avoid FODMAPs for two weeks. If your condition has improved, start Phase 4. If you are still having GI problems you will need to further restrict your foods by eliminating most food groups.

Eliminate Most Foods. At this point you should be trying this diet under the care of a physician, even though this very restrictive way of eating is only for seven to fourteen days. Authorities recommend different food lists, but the common denominator is that the foods on the list are least likely to generate gastrointestinal symptoms. Such foods include:

- wild cold-water fish like salmon or cod
- organic turkey, chicken, or lamb
- butternut squash, carrots, sweet potatoes, zucchini, parsnips, beets, bok choy
- olive oil, sea salt
- maple syrup (real!)
- avocados

---

2. Gerard E. Mullin and Kathie Madonna Swift, *The Inside Tract* (New York: Rodale, 2011), 180–191.

Eat only foods that do not cause GI upset, even if that means repeating some foods daily. Check in frequently with your doctor. Stay well hydrated. If you are at this stage, Dr. Gerard Mullin's book, *The Inside Tract*, contains extremely useful information as well as recipes for those who are trying an elimination diet, even if you are in a less restrictive phase.

By day seven of this phase, your gut should have healed sufficiently for you to start reintroducing foods in Phase 4.

Phase 4—Add Back

In the Add-Back Phase, you can start introducing foods back into your diet one by one. Under no circumstances should you reintroduce a food that has caused severe or anaphylactic reaction. If in doubt, leave it out! Depending on how many foods you have eliminated and are trying to add back, this phase can take weeks to months.

Keep eating the way you have been during the last phase you were in and choose a food to test. Note the food in your food diary. We suggest choosing a food that only gave you mild symptoms previously. Start in the morning, and call this Day 1. Dr. Mullin recommends simply placing the food in your mouth for few minutes, then taking it out to see if you develop any symptoms of inflammation over the next thirty minutes. Such symptoms would include rash, itching, or a runny nose. If symptoms occur, write them down and put an X beside that food on your list. You still need to avoid it. If you do not have any symptoms, eat a small amount to start, say a couple of teaspoons. Then, midday, eat a larger amount, about one-quarter cup. Note any symptoms. If none occur, then in the evening you can eat one-half cup.

If there is no reaction on Day 1, do not eat any more of the test food on Day 2 and Day 3. If there are no symptoms, you can add that food back into your diet. If you are unclear as to whether any symptoms occurred, then eat the same test food on Day 4, just more of it. See what happens. If there are no symptoms, you can incorporate that food again. If you have symptoms, avoid that food for several more months and then try to reintroduce it again.

One by one, add foods back in this fashion, keeping your test days at least three days apart. Even if you still need to avoid some foods, try again in three to six months. Over time, with a nutritious diet and the addition of the recommendations we are about to discuss, you will more than likely be able to enjoy a wide variety of foods without discomfort.

FOUR PHASE ELIMINATION DIET

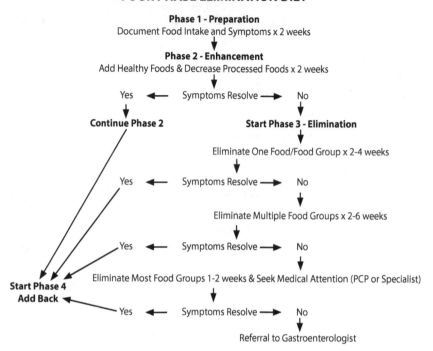

Phase 1 - Preparation
Document Food Intake and Symptoms x 2 weeks
↓
Phase 2 - Enhancement
Add Healthy Foods & Decrease Processed Foods x 2 weeks
↓
Yes ← Symptoms Resolve → No

Continue Phase 2   **Start Phase 3 - Elimination**

Eliminate One Food/Food Group x 2-4 weeks
↓
Yes ← Symptoms Resolve → No

Eliminate Multiple Food Groups x 2-6 weeks
↓
Yes ← Symptoms Resolve → No

Eliminate Most Food Groups 1-2 weeks & Seek Medical Attention (PCP or Specialist)
↓
**Start Phase 4
Add Back** ←   Yes ← Symptoms Resolve → No

Referral to Gastroenterologist

ELIMINATION DIET
Phase 1—Preparation

		Sunday	Monday	Tuesday	Wednesday	Thursday	Friday	Saturday
Waking until Lunch	Food							
	Symptoms							
Lunch until Dinner	Food							
	Symptoms							
Dinner until Bedtime	Food							
	Symptoms							

Probiotics, Prebiotics, and Digestive Enzymes

Probiotics are foods that contain beneficial bacteria that aid in digestion. Probiotic foods are fermented foods like yogurt, sauerkraut, kimchi, and miso. These foods maintain a healthy balance of "good' bacteria in your gut and discourage the growth of bacteria that threaten your digestive health.

Prebiotics are foods that promote the growth of the beneficial bacteria in your colon. Think of prebiotics as foods that your "good" bacteria like to eat. The interesting thing about prebiotics is that they pass through your stomach and small intestine undigested. When they arrive in your colon, your "good" bacteria process the prebiotics by fermenting them. This results in the creation of the short chain fatty acids (SCFAs) we discussed previously. Recall that SCFAs are vital in maintaining colon health, preventing colon cancer, and decreasing inflammation. Prebiotics improve digestion and the function of your immune system. They also increase absorption of minerals from all the food you eat.

Examples of prebiotics are:
- almonds
- asparagus
- garlic
- greens (beet, mustard, and turnip, among others)
- leeks
- oats
- onions
- sweet potato

Ideally, probiotics and prebiotics are present and plentiful in the foods you are eating and your natural digestive enzymes are functioning well. Unfortunately, this is not always the case and supplementation may be required. If you are already have digestive problems, eating a lot of fermented foods or those that contain prebiotics can cause bloating, gas, and diarrhea. If your digestive enzyme production is weak or the enzymes don't function properly, you cannot break down your food efficiently and gastrointestinal symptoms will arise. If you are noticing this correlation, speak to your healthcare provider about temporarily using commercial probiotics and prebiotics along with digestive enzymes. Continue to adjust your diet slowly. As your gut heals, you will be able to better tolerate these healthy foods and decrease your reliance on supplements.

Stress Management

So many of the most difficult-to-solve conditions in gastroenterology appear to be due to an exaggerated response or imbalance in the gut-brain-microbiome axis. We spoke at length about the interconnectedness of this system in chapter 2. In this section we would like to spend a little more time addressing chronic stress and why it is a major influence on your gastrointestinal health. Understanding how chronic stress can lead to gut dysfunction and damage your health may give you added impetus to make changes.

Your gut is exquisitely sensitive to your emotional state and your emotional state is influenced by your internal and external environment. Everything that happens to you, everything you see, say, do, or even think can change your emotions and subsequently your stress levels. Maybe you had to sleep less or work harder to accomplish a goal. Perhaps you lost your job or got a promotion. You may have married, divorced, or lost a loved one. All these events may require you to use more of your resources—your time, your money, your strength. These events are considered stressors. We have not even discussed environmental stressors such as pollution and overcrowding; societal stressors such as racism, gender bias, and poverty; and catastrophic stressors such as war, violence, and abuse. The word "stress" often has a negative connotation, but even normally joyful events such as the birth of a baby can be stressful.

When you live through these stressful life events, changes occur in all aspects of your physiology. This "gearing up" to face the increased demands on your metabolism, intellect, or psyche has been referred to as "allostasis," meaning "achieving stability through change."[3] These

---

3. P. Sterling and J. Ever, "Allostasis: A New Paradigm to Explain Arousal Pathology," in *Handbook of Life Stress, Cognition, and Health*, eds. S. Fisher and J. Reason (New York: John Wiley and Sons, 1988), 629–649.

stressors could be good, tolerable, or toxic. Whether "good" or "bad," the cumulative effects of such stressors are referred to as the "allostatic load."[4] Under usual circumstances, this state of heightened functioning resolves, and your immune, endocrine, and nervous systems are taken off high alert. Ordinarily, we are able to cope with these periods of allostasis, especially if we have been attentive to the needs of our bodies and minds, staying healthy, active, and well rested. This is much like topping up your bank account, saving for the proverbial rainy day.

But not everyone has the same reserves. Your fiscal, physical, or emotional state can vary throughout your life. Sometimes uncontrollable events occur one on top of the other. Sometimes we simply do not take the time or make the effort to care for ourselves as we know we should. Whatever the reason, when stressors overwhelm your resources, the body and mind are unable to return to a state of homeostasis, or balance. In this condition, dysregulation of the immune, endocrine, and nervous system occurs. Essentially, you get "stuck" in overdrive. This is called "allostatic overload," and it can create havoc.[5] Prolonged exposure to abnormal levels of immune modulators, hormones, and neurotransmitters results in physical changes throughout the body. This can lead to chronic inflammation and chronic diseases such as gastrointestinal and metabolic problems, heart disease, autoimmune conditions, pain syndromes, and psychological conditions. In the brain, exposure to the biochemical profile produced by allostatic overload can actually change its structure. Three brain regions affected by such toxic stress are the hippocampus, the amygdala, and the prefrontal cortex. These areas communicate with each other and modulate cognitive function, fear, aggression, and self-regulation. The interaction among these three regions also plays a part in turning on and turning off the neural and endocrine systems' response to stress.

The hippocampus is involved in memory of daily events, special memory, and mood regulation. The prefrontal cortex deals with decision-making, working memory, and self-regulatory behaviors such as mood and

---

4. B. S. McEwen, "Central Role of the Brain in Stress and Adaptation: Allostasis, Biological Embedding, and Cumulative Change," in *Stress: Concepts, Cognition, Emotion, and Behavior, Handbook of Stress Series*, vol. 1, ed. G. Fink (New York: Elsevier, 2016), 39–55.

5. McEwan, 43.

impulse control. Both of these structures help shut off the stress response, but under prolonged allostatic overload, the brain cells in these regions shrink and some of the connections between other brain cells are lost, allowing the chemical mediators of toxic stress to continue.

In contrast, the amygdala is the portion of the brain responsible for the autonomic nervous system's response to memories and emotions, particularly involving fear, anxiety, and aggression. Under chronic stress, the cells in the amygdala enlarge and create more connections among other brain cells, further driving the physical and emotional aspects of the fight-or-flight response. The amygdala turns on stress hormones and causes a variety of organ responses. In the gut, this can cause a sudden increase in motility leading to diarrhea. It can also cause nausea and vomiting. The body is trying to rid itself of gastric and intestinal contents. Digestion is not an important function when under siege. However, making glucose available for energy production is vital if you are preparing to fight or flee. So this same stress response causes an elevation in blood sugar, which is detrimental to a diabetic if it occurs constantly.

By understanding how the architecture of the brain changes under chronic stress, you can see how difficult it can be to recover from a period of extreme stress. It is as though the nervous system is locked in this abnormal physiological state. The nervous system in this sense includes the brain, the gut, and the microbiome. Recall that these three entities are intricately connected.

It is tempting to rely solely on medications to alleviate chronic stress, but numerous studies cite the effectiveness of the concurrent use of other interventions to achieve this goal. Although there are many possible approaches to stress reduction, two of the most effective and easily accessible are physical activity and meditation. These activities can dampen the "fight-or-flight" response and modulate the neuroendocrine-immune system to restore normal organ function. By using effective treatments from both Eastern and Western traditions, you can create prompt and long-lasting improvements in your gastrointestinal health. Let's look at these interventions with respect to stress management and digestive health.

Physical Activity. When you keep your body moving with activities you enjoy, you initiate a host of biochemical, hormonal, and neurological changes that bring your sympathetic and parasympathetic nervous systems back into balance. This alleviates stress and improves your mood. We will be discussing movement as medicine in the remainder of this chapter as well as in chapters 4 and 5. Even if you do not have diabetes or weight problems, we encourage you to read these chapters for additional information about the benefits of physical activity.

Meditation: Regulation of the breath has been used for millennia to calm the mind and heal the body. Even without a modern understanding of how the brain and body communicate, the ancients formulated breathing techniques that balanced the autonomic nervous system. This is the part of your brain, nerves, immune, and endocrine systems that determines your state of relaxation. The autonomic nervous system is composed of the sympathetic nervous system and the parasympathetic nervous system. The sympathetic nervous system initiates the release of stress hormones when your brain perceives that you are in danger. These hormones cause your heart rate to elevate, raise your blood pressure, and make glucose available to fuel your muscles in preparation for combat or evasive maneuvers. It can also cause your bowels to empty and your stomach to eject its contents. This reaction is known as the fight-or-flight response. In contrast, the parasympathetic nervous system calms all these processes and returns the body to a normal state of activity. Slow, deep breathing stimulates the main nerve of the parasympathetic nervous system called the vagus nerve, which in turn releases hormones and neurotransmitters that slow your heart rate, lower your blood pressure, resume normal bowel function, and generally bring your body into balance.[6]

As we saw in chapter 1, meditation, which often makes use of breath control, has many important benefits, both physical and psychological. You can meditate anytime and anywhere during the day. It can be five minutes, ten minutes, or twenty minutes, depending on how much time you have. Even a ten-minute meditation break during work can be beneficial—like taking a mini-vacation. You just need to make time to do it. No matter how

---

6. T. M. Srinivasan, "Pranayama and Brain Correlates," *Ancient Science of Life* 11, no. 1-2: 1–6; D. Krshnakumar, M. R. Hamblin, and S. Lakshmanan, "Meditation and Yoga Can Modulate Brain Mechanisms That Affect Behaviour and Anxiety," *Ancient Science of Life* 2, no. 1: 13–19, https://doi.org/10.14259/as/v2i2il1.171; Michael M. Zanoni, "Healing Resonance Qi Gong and Hamanaleo Meditation," https://www.mikezanoni.com/meditation-qi-gong, accessed February 4, 2018.

much you know, it is not useful without practice. Some people say you have to meditate thirty to forty-five minutes to get results. This can be intimidating for busy people; they won't do it, because they don't have forty-five minutes. You can take less time to meditate but do it more often and do it correctly; you can still get the benefits. It is better than not doing it at all. If you have never practiced meditation, here are some methods for you to try.

Position. Your body position should be very comfortable. You can be standing, sitting, or even lying on the ground; just do whatever feels most comfortable. If you prefer to sit on the floor, you may need a cushion or pillow to help your posture so you won't have backache during meditation. If you choose to lie on the floor, you may fall asleep during meditation practice. This is because meditation makes you very comfortable and relaxed.

Mind. During meditation practice, some say you need to remove all thoughts from your mind. This is actually impossible. Neuroscience has shown us that when you are awake, your brain is always on idle. If you think about it from an evolutionary perspective, this makes perfect sense. Your brain is always alert, always thinking, and ready to react to any danger that may arise. This constant brain activity has been dubbed the Default Mode Network. It is like the program that is supposed to be running in the background of your mind. As you are meditating, random thoughts will float in and out of your consciousness. This is normal and happens to everyone; it does not mean you have failed. Expect this to happen and when it does, notice the thought and return your attention to your breathing.

First, your mind should focus on your breathing: how deep, how slow, and how even it is. In the beginning, your breath may be too fast, but as you continue your daily practice, you will realize you can breathe more deeply, more slowly, and with more intention.

Next, focus on total relaxation. Ask yourself some questions: are my shoulders relaxed? Is my neck relaxed? Is my back relaxed? Is my body comfortable? Make sure your answer to each is yes. If not, relax each part of the body at each exhalation until all parts of the body are relaxed.

You are meditating now, so it is not the right time for you to think of work. Your mind never leaves your body, no matter how many things you have to deal with. When you leave meditation, you can do whatever you need to do. But during meditation practice, we focus on *now*.

Breath. Focus on breaths that are deep, slow, mindful, and controlled. With each inhalation, you bring maximum oxygen to your body; with each exhalation you relax your entire body. Really pay attention to your breath. A very effective and simple way to achieve this state of relaxation is to exhale for about twice as long as you inhale. This technique will further activate the parasympathetic nervous system and improve digestive function.

Body. Your body needs to be in a comfortable position. If you are not comfortable, you will need to find a way to make yourself comfortable. Your body needs to be completely relaxed from head to toe, including the fingers. Your facial muscles also need to be relaxed, including your jaw. Place your tongue behind your upper teeth, on the upper palate, which keeps the roof of your mouth open.

When you finish your meditation, you will feel much better, much calmer, and much more relaxed. You will feel less stressed and more focused. You can achieve more if you remain calm and focused, mindful of your feelings and thoughts as you integrate new therapies or foods into your life.

Before we discuss specific interventions, we would like to add a few words about Daoism. We feel that this approach to living helps to alleviate chronic stress and thereby improve digestive function. As we discussed earlier, Dao (sometimes spelled "Tao") means the Way, or following what is most natural, alive, and spontaneous. Its guiding principle is to follow what is natural so that your own inner nature will effortlessly unfold. Everyone unfolds in different ways. The only person you need to follow is yourself; you do whatever is right for you. Many Buddhists, Christians, and Sufis study and practice the Dao because it helps ground the spirit into the body. The Daoist principles of qi, the life force, are in all creatures. They are based on balancing the receptive and expressive, or yin and yang, forces that resonate within everybody, every society, and every atom of nature. Thus, the original duality of being and nonbeing is mirrored in the dualities of the physical world. If one thing is difficult, there must be something else that is easy by comparison. One of the keys to Daoist thought is the recognition of dualities. This is the yin and the yang.

All processes have active and passive principles. All physical conditions contain interdependent opposites, but many people think of these dualities as mutually exclusive. Instead of seeing active and passive parts of action as complements, we label one as good and make the other bad, and try to ignore or eliminate the "bad." Often, there is no absolute right and wrong; it depends on the situation. The more we understand this philosophy, the better we deal with our life stress.

The Dao is a beautiful path for everyday life and everyone who chooses to walk on it. It is simple, mild, smooth, soothing, pure, and still—yet it is also moving and present. It is in everything and has unbreakable power. The Dao is the way that has no end, and learning its wisdom helps us to grow and be happy.

The Dao teaches us to flow with nature and not against nature; to be plain and simple; to desire less and be satisfied with what we have; to walk on the path without analyzing the path; to be humble, gentle, and easy; and to be simultaneously empty and full. This way we will be able to handle stress better at work and home, untangle our minds, and live peacefully.

Now, moving from theory to practice, we discuss specific Eastern modalities that can be used on your healing journey to achieve optimal digestive health.

Healing with Chinese Herbal Medicine

Healers from all traditions have used plants to treat gastrointestinal disorders for centuries upon centuries. Many Chinese herbal formulas that are in use today have been used to treat digestive problems for thousands of years. The fact that these formulas are still prescribed is a testament to their utility.

As tempting as it may be to order a Chinese herbal formula over the Internet based on a description of symptoms in an advertisement, we discourage this approach. Herbs are drugs. Just as food has medicinal properties, so too do herbs. The majority of Western pharmaceuticals are derived from plants, so it should come as no surprise that herbs could have side effects if taken incorrectly or in conjunction with incompatible herbs, foods, or drugs. Purchasing herbal formulas off the Internet or sharing someone else's herbs is highly discouraged. Before a practitioner of Eastern medicine prescribes an herbal formula, a lot of information is gathered from the patient to ensure optimal outcomes with minimal adverse effects.

Chinese herbs are used in various combinations, unlike Western herbs and medications, which are generally used individually. These herbal formulas are elegantly constructed, creating combinations that enhance the actions of each component and, at the same time, minimize possible side effects. In Chinese herbal prescriptions, different combinations of herbs influence the function of the organ-channel energy networks in the body.

In Eastern medicine, the organs are described as being associated with specific channels. These pairs of organs and channels create energy networks that have particular functions. Chinese herbal medicine is effective in balancing these energetic networks, harmonizing the body and the mind. In Western terms, this is akin to using pharmaceuticals to modulate organ physiology.

Herbal formulas can be cooked by the patient from raw herbs prescribed by the practitioner, reconstituted from granules and sipped as a tea, or taken in pill form. Pills or tablets are easier to take, but may not be as potent as cooked herbs or teas. Sometimes a patient is started on cooked herbs and then transitioned to pills for maintenance.

Regardless of the formulation, the most important aspect of herbal therapy is making the correct diagnosis within the paradigm of Eastern medicine. Only then can the correct formula be prescribed. For this reason, patients should consult a qualified professional herbalist who is trained in Eastern medicine. In Eastern healing, even though several people can have the same Western diagnosis, such as irritable bowel syndrome, gastroesophageal reflux disease, or another ailment, the best herbal formula for each of those people may be different. Everyone has a different constitution. Some patients have an inherent vulnerability in one or more organ systems. In Eastern medicine this is referred to as a weakness or excess of organ energy.

Herbal formulas can be used in conjunction with other Eastern healing modalities such as acupuncture, tui na (Chinese massage), meditation, qigong, and taiji. Also, appropriate dietary changes and exercise will help speed your recovery. Ideally, as your condition improves, your reliance on herbs may diminish. You may find that consistent attention to healthy food choices; persistent cultivation of your meditation, qigong and taiji practice; and using acupuncture or tui na as needed will help you maintain normal digestive function. At that point, you can consult with your Eastern practitioner about diminishing or discontinuing your herbal formula. Similarly, if you are taking Western medications, you can speak to your doctor about modifying your regimen.

Remember that everyone is different. Some people must take herbs or medications for a longer time than others, but incorporating all these recommended healing practices will increase the likelihood of long-lasting results.

Healing with Acupuncture and Tui Na (Chinese Massage)

From an Eastern perspective, acupuncture is an effective treatment for a "tune-up" of the organ-channel system. It reduces the excesses, supports the weaknesses, and promotes a smooth flow of energy within the body. Tui na (Chinese deep massage) has similar effects. Tui na therapy can also be used in conjunction with herbs and acupuncture to unblock the stagnant qi and promote circulation.

Western science has determined that acupuncture modulates the nervous system, causing biochemical, hormonal, and neurological changes that normalize the functioning of the digestive system. Acupuncture has been shown to decrease abdominal pain, nausea, and vomiting. Acupuncture treatments can also regulate the speed of peristalsis and has been used to correct both diarrhea and constipation.[7] Acupuncture is also excellent for decreasing stress by balancing the autonomic nervous system. It has been used effectively to treat anxiety, depression, and post-traumatic stress disorder.

Both acupuncture and Chinese massage may involve multiple visits, depending on the severity of your symptoms. Either method can greatly enhance healing results if you combine acupuncture and tui na with taiji or qigong practice.

---

7. T. Takahashi, "Mechanism of Acupuncture on Neuromodulation in the Gut— A Review," *Neuromodulation* 14, no. 1 (Jan. 2011): 8–12, https://doi.org/10.111/j.1525-1403.2010.00295.x.

Both modalities can be very effective when you find well-trained and experienced practitioners; however, if after several weeks of treatment you do not feel any improvement, we suggest that you return to your primary care provider for further evaluation. You may also choose to seek out another Eastern practitioner. Just as there are variations among Western practitioners, there are also differences in skill and expertise among Eastern practitioners. Do not deprive yourself of the healing aspects of acupuncture or tui na if your first treatments are not successful. Acupuncture and Chinese massage work very well for sufferers of mild and moderate depression and anxiety. For severe symptoms, you should be treated with both Eastern and Western medicine. Where you sit on the continuum of emotional well-being can shift quickly, so it is wise to involve both your Eastern and Western healthcare providers.

Healing with Taiji and Qigong

Taiji and qigong are ancient methods of healing that incorporate movement, breath control, and meditation. Taiji, more accurately called *taijiquan* in Chinese culture, is a martial art that has been known for centuries for its health benefits, including psychological benefits. Now, since the world has recognized its healing benefits, more and more people practice taiji all over the world. Taiji is a higher level of qi practice, or some say a "higher-level qigong." Both taiji and qigong are excellent methods for reducing anxiety, depression, and sleep difficulties. For beginners, starting with qigong is a good idea. For this reason, we focus on qigong and have devoted a whole chapter to this discussion (chapter 6). In the paragraphs that follow, we introduce some concepts about taiji and qigong.

Practicing taiji and qigong helps us stay in the present moment. When you are practicing taiji, your mind is focused on learning and moving with controlled energy. Once you learn to stay in the present, you automatically detach from the "monkey mind." The term monkey mind is the label attached to your internal voice, the voice you hear in your mind that constantly chatters in the background as you go about your day.

Over time, by practicing taiji or qigong, you will learn to be aware of the monkey mind but not to react to its narrative. You will feel calm, peaceful, centered, and grounded (rooted). You may feel a smooth flow of the qi (energy); you may become more positive, physically and mentally stronger, and better able to face negative situations with ease. You eventually will be able to shift your energy. Other benefits of practicing taiji and qigong are improved digestion and metabolism, improved sexual functioning, increased blood circulation and cardiovascular fitness, increased youthfulness, and increased longevity.

Taiji and qigong practice consists of smoothing energy flow, letting go of negative thoughts, and becoming more positive and open to all. Both taiji and qigong come from Daoist practice and involve balance and nature. All movements entail the yin and yang: constantly shifting weight and turning the waist; left and right, up and down, empty and full, stillness and movement, mind and body, breathing in and breathing out.

Problems in the gut can be exacerbated by emotional imbalance caused by situations like unresolved past experiences and unmanaged, ongoing stress. From an Eastern medical perspective we would say that these emotional imbalances cause your qi to stagnate. Simply put, qi is not flowing the way it is supposed to flow. Qi flow can be affected by such factors as genetics, long-term use of certain medications and long-term misuse of alcohol or other harmful substances. The practice of taiji and qigong have a positive influence on both emotional and qi balance. The movements and patterns of breathing focus and calm the mind and promote the smooth flow of energy in the body. The key is regular practice.

Because the movements involved in qigong are concise and simple to learn, we recommend developing a qigong practice first. For qigong exercises to help alleviate gastrointestinal and emotional distress, please see chapter 6.

Qigong has several important characteristics.
- It is easy to learn, easy to remember, and easy to practice.
- It empowers the mind, strengthens the body, and improves stamina and self-esteem.
- Its symmetrical movements balance both sides of the brain to harmonize brain activity.

- The movements involve learning that stimulates brain functions.
- The slow and balanced movements calm and balance the brain neurotransmitters, acting as a "natural tranquilizer."
- The gentle physical movement enhances energy flow in the body and improves daily energy levels.
- The localized steps require a small space to practice and can be practiced indoors when the weather is inclement.
- The coordinated, soothing movements improve coordination and balance, open energy channels, and help you open up to nature when practicing outdoors.
- Most movements are slow, soothing, calming, graceful, peaceful, and especially suitable for the older generation and those with chronic illness. Therefore it is regarded as the best healing exercise.

How does qigong help with digestive problems?

1. Learning. Learning is a big part of healing, especially in the healing of emotions. We know our emotions influence our physical body. The brain's emotional center needs to be refreshed, nourished, stimulated, and balanced. When you learn things you are not familiar with, you start to shift your focus onto new knowledge, new approaches, and a new life. This sort of internal transformation can improve your situation in life. It is as if you are shifting negative energy to positive energy. The more positive energy you have, the better the chance you can be healed. Once you focus on learning qigong and then start to practice diligently, your qigong form will become more graceful and beautiful. This gives you a feeling of accomplishment and satisfaction. No matter how old you are, learning can always benefit your physical and emotional health.

2. Specific and Balanced Movements. Qigong is very soothing and relaxing, and has open-framed movements that help open the energy channels. The movements are symmetrical to harmonize both hemispheres of the brain. It is like a natural tranquilizer that immediately calms your mind and your body. The brain has two hemispheres, which carry out different functions. Most people are dominant on one side or the other of their brains: some people are strong in language, whereas others are strong in artistic expression. Some people learn certain things quickly and other things slowly. If you overuse the dominant side of the brain throughout your life and fail to use the minor side of your brain, that side may become understimulated and an imbalance can occur. Qigong exercise balances both sides of the brain so you develop a well-balanced brain, improving cognitive skills, communication skills, social skills, and so on.

3. Smooth Qi (Energy) Flow in the Body. Qi is vital energy, or life force. It is the energy that underlies everything in the universe. Qi in the human body refers to the various types of bioenergy associated with human health and vitality. Qi controls the functioning of all parts of the body.

4. Group Energy. Human beings are social beings. Qigong practice brings out a great deal of group energy and is most often practiced in group settings, either in a classroom or outdoors. This method of practice fosters discussion, friendship, and all the positive benefits of group energy. Because the energy of each individual affects the energy of others during practice, everyone feels good.

5. Martial Arts Applications. In qigong, some of the movements have some martial relevance. People choose to practice qigong for different reasons, such as for inner peace, healing, martial training or self-defense, relief of stress, longevity, maintaining good health, or disease prevention, for flexibility, and for increasing energy and stamina. Qigong and martial arts predate taiji. Compared with qigong, more of the movements in taiji have a martial art aspect and can be used for self-defense. The martial arts movements found in qigong and taiji make you feel stronger, especially internally.

Other Self-Healing Practices

Be Physically Active. Whether your practice is Western or Eastern, daily movement is important. You can choose jogging, walking, running, swimming, tennis, ball games, hiking, taiji, qigong, martial arts, aerobic exercise, ballroom dancing, yoga—whatever you enjoy. Remember that any sort of regular movement counts. Even mopping your floors, dusting your ceiling fans, and dancing around your living room are examples of movements that can improve your digestion and metabolism. It has been shown that exercise can benefit the gut-brain-microbiome axis by increasing the diversity of the microbiome in a way that favors the beneficial bacteria that produce serotonin, which improves mood, and short chain fatty acids, which decrease inflammation. It is important you find an activity you actually enjoy. Studies in rodents show that allowing mice to voluntary run on the wheel in their cage yielded the beneficial results previously mentioned, but if the mice were forced to run, the exercise had a negative effect, decreasing the numbers of beneficial bacteria and decreasing bacterial diversity.[8]

Practice Being Positive. It is not easy to be positive all the time, but it can be done with practice. Developing resilience and optimism can help manage the stress of chronic illness. We have seen many patients who heal at different rates. The main difference in their healing is their attitude; the way they think influences how they act. People who are more positive heal faster than those who are negative.

Avoid Overanalyzing. There are major differences between Western psychology and Daoist healing. Western psychology is constantly analyzing, searching out the reasons for everything. This may lead to an understanding of the cause of a problem but not how to get rid of it.

In Daoist healing and Daoist psychology, we practice letting go. We accept that things are not always fair and not everything can be reasoned out. Do we have to know the "why" of everything? No. When we are able to let go, we feel like we just unloaded five hundred pounds off our shoulders. This may not always be easy, but it can be done with mindful practice. When you are able to let go, your spirit and energy are lifted right way.

Some people worry about things that may never happen, which is a complete waste of energy. Cautiousness is good when dealing with unexpected situations. But being overcautious, worrying too much, and being always nervous create negativity and blockage in the mind and loss of enjoyment of life.

People who think too much, worry too much, plan too much, and fear too much can create stress and tension, which trigger negative emotions that adversely impact their gut.

---

8. Alyssa Dalton, Christine Mermier, and Micha Zuhl, "Exercise Influence on the Microbiome-Gut-Brain Axis," *Gut Microbes* 10, no. 5 (2019): 555–568, https://doi.org/10.1080/19490976.2018.1562268.

We cannot control everything that can happen or that has happened in the past. We cannot predict everything that may happen in the future. We can only be prepared, try to manage our current situation to the best of our ability, and live in the moment. Overanalyzing is a waste of energy. It's better to preserve our energy for the important things like striving for better health, happiness, and well-being. Then, when bad things happen, we will always find ways to deal with them.

Practice Forgiveness. Forgiving is a good healing practice. Too often we hold onto slights and grudges, keeping the negative energy within us. This negativity can be held within the body, and the gut is a prime target given the relationship between the enteric and central nervous systems.

Forgiveness creates positive energy and helps us to let go with ease. When we forgive, we feel free, open, happy, and relaxed. There also seems to be a connection between the capacity to forgive and chronic pain. Those who cannot forgive another person are more likely to be troubled by chronic pain or have a low tolerance for pain.[9]

Even when we have truly been wronged we benefit from forgiving the offender. To be clear, forgiving someone for an egregious act is not the same thing as excusing them. We all make some mistakes in our lives, and we all learn from mistakes. If we forgive, love grows. Love can reinforce forgiveness, and forgiveness can nurture love. They go hand in hand. Hate is the opposite. It creates negative energy and is an obstacle to healing.

"True forgiveness includes total acceptance. And out of acceptance, wounds are healed and happiness is possible again."

—Catherine Marshall, American author

Be with the Dao. We have learned about the Dao, and now it is time to practice. Let's be more natural and spontaneous; let's be more relaxed, accepting, tolerant, appreciative, and positive.

Chinese people have used Daoism for centuries. They use Daoism in almost every area of life to find the right solution to their own needs. Daoism does not directly tell you what to do, but it does give you direction to help you to see things more clearly. It teaches you to unload your burdens,

---

9. S. O'Beime, A. M. Katsimigos, and D. Harmon, "Forgiveness and Chronic Pain: A Systematic Review," *Irish Journal of Medical Science* (Mar. 3, 2020), https://doi.org/10.1007/s11845-020-02200-y.

free your mind, and let things happen spontaneously and naturally. Over-reacting to people or situations can cause conflict. If you stay focused, calm, and nonjudgmental, you can resolve many problems and overcome many obstacles. If you go against the natural flow, on the other hand, you may make things worse; healing needs the natural flow.

With Daoist study and practice, you can be happy no matter whether you are rich or poor, what your intellectual level or occupation are, or how old you are.

Be Patient. Healing takes time. Don't get discouraged or frustrated if you don't feel better immediately. Time allows you to learn, heal, find happiness, and achieve your goals. Be patient, but don't waste time; use it wisely to create the environment you need to nourish your spirit.

Focus on the Present. Staying focused on the present is a tough thing for many people. Our minds are always active and busy. We have so many distractions in our lives. The busier we are, the more stress we tend to have. We get preoccupied by pressing work deadlines, raising children, maintaining houses, paying bills, investing money, and planning for vacations and retirement. All these tasks are important and deserve attention, but often we try to do everything at once. We try to multitask. When we are doing more than one thing, our mind is in a different place. The commotion of the day can even appear in our dreams when we are sleeping.

In order to be productive and accomplish our work with less stress, we need to focus on the present—on whatever we are doing at this moment. This is mindfulness.

Get a Good Night's Sleep. No matter how stressful your day has been, do whatever you can to ensure a good night's sleep. In chapter 2, we discussed the connection between sleep and digestive health. In one of our previous books, *True Wellness: The Mind* we went into greater detail about normal and abnormal sleep patterns, external factors that influence sleep, and strategies for improving the quality and quantity of your sleep to restore energy and enhance healing. Ideally, you need at least seven hours of restorative sleep each night and, as we discussed, it is extremely helpful to your digestion if your sleep coincides with usual day-night cycles.

By now, you have gained an even greater appreciation of the complexity of the digestive system and its influence on all aspects of your health.

We encourage you to explore some of the many excellent books we have listed in the Recommended Reading and Resources section for a more in-depth discussion of conventional medical approaches to gut health.

If you also suffer from diabetes or weight problems, continue on to chapters 4 and 5.

If gastrointestinal problems are your only concern, you can skip to chapter 6 to learn more about qigong and how to start your healing practice.

The True Wellness Approach to Digestive Problems

- Start the Four Phase Elimination Diet.
- Consider the use of probiotic, prebiotic, and digestive enzyme supplements if needed.
- Incorporate more movement into your daily life and strive to be active most days of the week.
- Decrease stress by using techniques such as meditation, taiji, and qigong.
- Find a reputable acupuncturist and receive regular treatments.
- If herbal formulas are recommended, ensure that your acupuncturist checks for possible drug/herb interactions and discuss the addition of herbs with your doctor.
- Follow your doctor's recommendations regarding medications and do not make dose adjustments without her knowledge.

CHAPTER 4

The True Wellness Approach to Diabetes

NINETY PERCENT OF DIABETES in the U.S. today is classified as type 2. Also, more the 90 percent of type-2 diabetics are overweight or obese. As little as a 5 percent loss of total body weight can help to control this disease.[1] If you are a type-2 diabetic or an overweight type-1 diabetic, we encourage you to read chapter 5 for a more in-depth approach to manage your diabetes through lifestyle changes that can lead to weight loss.

Type-2 diabetes arises primarily from insulin resistance, so the approach that Western medicine has taken in dealing with this epidemic is to target factors that lead to this condition. As we discussed in Chapter 2, one of the main factors leading to insulin resistance is chronic inflammation. A great deal of research has shown that improved diet and increasing exercise will decrease chronic inflammation, improve glucose control, and decrease complications related to the disease.

Diet

Since chronic inflammation is so frequently related to the onset of type-2 diabetes, a healthful diet is vital for successful management of this condition. You cannot think of this as a diet that you will only follow for a few weeks or months. You must find a new way of eating that will last a lifetime. This is actually simpler than it sounds.

---

1. American Society for Metabolic and Bariatric Surgery, "Type-2 Diabetes and Obesity: Twin Epidemics," https://asmbs.org/resources/weight-and-type-2-diabetes-after-bariatric-surgery-fact-sheet.

After writing his best-selling book *The Omnivore's Dilemma* that described various methods of food production in America, author Michael Pollan was besieged with correspondence asking him what is the healthiest possible way to eat. This prompted him to do further research and in his next book, *In Defense of Food*, Mr. Pollan proposed these three rules for a healthy diet:[2]

1. Eat food (meaning whole, unprocessed, non-synthetic food)
2. Mostly plants
3. Not too much

While an entirely vegetarian diet has many health benefits, most people find this to be a very difficult shift in lifestyle. Others feel unwell if they don't eat enough protein in the form of red meat, poultry, or fish. For this reason, many people have easily adopted Mr. Pollan's Three Rules by changing to the Mediterranean Diet. More recently, Dr. Mark Hyman, a leading medical authority, coined the term the "Pegan Diet." He combines small amounts of wild-caught or grass-fed animal protein, such as one would eat in a Paleo or ancestral diet, with whole-food, plant-based veganism. Hence, Dr. Hyman states that he is a Pegan. While Dr. Hyman invented this term primarily to poke fun at the vehemence of some Paleo and vegan friends, the description is apt.[3]

We have discussed the Mediterranean Diet and its benefits in decreasing chronic inflammation in our previous books in the True Wellness series and agree with Dr. Hyman that animal proteins, if eaten, should be of high quality and used in small portions. Veganism, Peganism, vegetarianism, and ancestral diets that minimize or avoid grains, are all similar to the Mediterranean diet in that the focus is on foods derived from plants. A plant-based diet will positively affect your microbiome and decrease chronic inflammation. Since there is a lot of research that has looked at the Mediterranean Diet and health outcomes, let's compare it to the way we typically eat.

---

2. Michael Pollan, *In Defense of Food* (New York: Penguin, 2008), 1.

3. Mark Hyman, MD, *Food: What the Heck Should I Eat?* (New York: Little, Brown Spark, 2018), 4.

The Standard American Diet (known in medical circles as the SAD Diet) is composed of large amounts of red meats, simple carbohydrates such as breads and pastas, and minimal fruits and vegetables. In contrast, the Mediterranean Diet minimizes red meat consumption to a few times per month and emphasizes the ingestion of fruits and vegetables to seven to ten times per day. Additionally, this diet includes daily portions of beans, legumes, and nuts. It substitutes olive oil instead of butter and other unhealthy fats. Fish and poultry are recommended at least twice weekly. Inclusion of wine is suggested on a daily basis. For those of you who do not or cannot use alcohol, the same health benefits can be achieved with grape juice.

Aside from the various recommendations of the Mediterranean Diet regarding meats, it seems that the cornerstone of its success is the emphasis on fruits and vegetables. Plants provide dozens and dozens of nutrients that aid in cell repair, improve metabolism, and even help prevent cancer. Most of us consider ourselves to be eating healthily if we consume two or three fruits or vegetables daily. It may seem onerous to add seven more portions, but the extra effort is well worth it. For example, in a study that included 1.5 million healthy adults it was shown that following a Mediterranean diet was associated with a reduced risk of dying of heart disease or cancer, and a reduced risk of getting cancer, Parkinson's, and Alzheimer's diseases. That's a pretty good incentive for eating your vegetables![4]

If your diabetes is not well controlled, your blood sugar levels will be persistently elevated. This leads to chronic inflammation. Inflammation causes cellular damage that slows down the normal metabolism.[5] Refined carbohydrates found in processed foods increases blood sugars very quickly after they are eaten and those sugars stay in the blood stream longer because, in the case of type-2 diabetes, your cells are not very responsive to insulin.

On the other hand, eating whole, unprocessed carbohydrates, like brown rice, bulgur wheat, and quinoa, slows down digestion and the

---

4. Mayo Clinic, "A Heart-Healthy Eating Plan," http://www.mayoclinic.com/health/mediterranean-diet/CL00011/NSECTIONGROUP=2, accessed Sept 16, 2012.

5. Antonio Ceriello, MD, PhD, "Diabetic Complications: From Oxidative Stress to Inflammatory Cardiovascular Disorders," http://www.medicographia.com/2011/07/diabetic-complications-from-oxidative-stress-to-inflammatory-cardiovascular-disorders/.

release of glucose and insulin into the bloodstream. The difference in the speed at which whole foods are digested is due to the increased amounts of fiber they contain: there is an inverse correlation between dietary fiber and oxidative stress with resulting inflammation. This means the more fiber you ingest, the less inflammation in your body. Fruits and vegetables are considered complex carbohydrates because they are essentially made of natural sugars: they are unprocessed and unrefined. They are beneficial for many reasons, not the least of which is the large amounts of fiber they contain.

Fruits, vegetables, and whole grains are the basis of an anti-inflammatory regimen. Not only will these foods supply large amounts of fiber, they also supply magnesium, zinc, B vitamins, vitamin E, and lignans, all of which help decrease inflammation.

So, how can you tell which foods will give a consistent, even release of glucose and won't overload your mitochondria? Check their glycemic load. You may have already heard of the glycemic index, a measure of how quickly a food is digested into simple sugars within a specific time. The glycemic load is similar, but it gives more information.

The glycemic index uses a standardized amount of white bread as its reference point because white bread is metabolized so quickly and causes striking increases in blood sugar levels after it is eaten; it is assigned a value of one hundred. Research has been done that compares how the same amount of other foods affect blood sugar levels in the same amount of time. The glycemic index of a food is assigned a number between one and one hundred based on how quickly it raises blood sugar values compared with white bread. For example, an apple has a low glycemic index value because it causes a lower rise in blood sugar levels compared with white bread in the same amount of time.

Glycemic load uses the glycemic index but goes a step further. It also takes into account the amount of carbohydrates a food contains in a typical serving. When you compare foods, you find that those foods with a low glycemic index will also have a low glycemic load, but those with a high glycemic index may go either way once the carbohydrate content is considered. Foods that have rapidly digestible sugar but also a high water content will have a high glycemic index value but a low glycemic load. This is because there is relatively little sugar in an average serving of the food.[6] Watermelon is a good example.

Using either the glycemic index or glycemic load values is a good way to choose foods that will reduce your risk of chronic disease due to inflammation. Using the glycemic load also has additional benefits. Research has shown that diets based on low-glycemic-load foods are easier to sustain and result in decreased food cravings, spontaneously smaller portion sizes, and increased weight loss.[7] (For a list of the glycemic index and glycemic load of common foods, please refer to the appendix.)

Exercise

Adequate exercise is essential to improving insulin utilization within the body. By exercising, you will improve insulin sensitivity in both fat cells and skeletal muscles. By increasing your muscle mass by including weight-lifting in your exercise program, you can raise your metabolic rate (the number of calories you burn at rest). This will decrease your body fat, triglyceride levels, and blood pressure.[8]

For those already taking insulin, better insulin sensitivity within your cells will result in a decrease in the amount of injected insulin required. You will begin to see your glucose readings improving as you are checking them throughout the day. You should consult with your doctor regarding food intake around exercise times to avoid hypoglycemia (glucose levels that are too low). Of course, any adjustment in your insulin regimen should be approved by your healthcare provider.

Supplements

A variety of minerals and vitamins have been shown to improve glucose tolerance, either by improving insulin production or sensitivity at the

---

6. Sarah K. Kahn, RD, MPH, PhD, "The Glycemic Index/Load," in *Integrative Medicine*, 3rd ed., ed. David Rakel, MD (Philadelphia: Saunders/Elsevier, 2012), 2287.

7. Kahn, 2288.

8. David Rakel, MD, "Insulin Resistance Syndrome" in *Integrative Medicine*, 1st ed., ed. David Rakel, MD, (Philadelphia: Saunders, Elsevier, 2003), 225.

cellular level. Omega 3 fatty acids act to decrease chronic inflammation, which can disrupt glucose metabolism. Such supplements include:

- chromium: 200–1000 mcg daily
- alpha-lipoic acid: 50–100 mg daily
- vitamin D: 1000–4000 units daily
- omega 3 fatty acids: 1–4 grams daily
- magnesium: 200–500mg/day

Botanicals

Some plants, either eaten whole or as extracts, are used in many cultures to improve blood sugars. It is important to let your healthcare provider know if you are using any such agent as it may have an impact on your medication dosage. It is equally important to inform your East Asian practitioner in case they are prescribing an herbal formula in order to avoid lowering your blood sugar too far. Some examples of botanicals that can be used are:

- cinnamon: 1–5 grams ground bark with meals or an equivalent amount of cinnamon extract
- pycnogenol: 100–200 mg daily
- panax ginseng extract: 100–400 mg daily

Mind-Body Exercises

Mind-body exercises that focus on decreasing stress are very useful in the management of diabetes. When people are stressed, their bodies release hormones such as epinephrine and cortisol that are designed to ready their bodies for physical activity such as fighting an enemy or running from a predator. This ancient physiological response provided a great survival mechanism by increasing glucose levels and preparing the body for sudden motion. In modern times, these same hormones are released in response to stress and blood sugars rise. By using relaxation techniques to decrease the levels of these hormones, blood sugars are similarly lowered.[9]

---

9. Victor S. Sierpina, MD, "Diabetes Mellitus" in *Integrative Medicine*, 1st ed., ed. David Rakel, MD, (Philadelphia: Saunders, Elsevier, 2003), 236.

Examples of such methods are biofeedback, meditation, and guided imagery. East Asian methods of moving mind-body techniques include taiji and qigong.

Natural Healing for Diabetes

No matter what illness you have, there is always a natural way to improve your condition. You may still need to use medications, but by adding natural therapies, you may need less. There are many other benefits to using natural methods, as we shall see.

If you have type-1 diabetes, you will need to continue your use of insulin to replace the insulin your pancreas cannot produce. There is no cure, yet. If it can be diagnosed very early while the person's pancreas can still make some of its own insulin, then natural methods may keep the pancreas working longer and decrease insulin requirements by supporting the function of the pancreas. It is a lifetime's work that takes effort, a positive mindset, and dedication. Anything is possible. If you don't try, you will not have the chance to see the possibilities.

For type-2 diabetes, natural methods work very well if you follow the healing principles and guidelines. This also takes effort and dedication. Medication to control blood sugar is effective but does not correct the underlying problems we discussed in chapter 2. The underlying problems can lead to other diseases beyond diabetes. Moreover, medications often carry complications you can avoid by using natural healing methods. But do not stop taking medication without consulting your doctor.

To be able to heal, first, you need to have an open mind and be open to natural methods and changing your habits. Second, you need to be willing to do some work yourself, such as changing your diet, practicing mindful eating, being active daily, reducing stress levels, balancing work and home schedule, and being persistent in the mindful practice of these natural methods. Natural healing involves self-care and belief in oneself. It is worth the investment because of the multiple benefits you will reap. Making the following lifestyle changes can not only control sugar metabolism, they can reduce chronic inflammation, prevent heart attack and stroke, prevent cancer, improve immune function, improve energy, and delay the aging process.

Natural Healing Methods

1. Diet

There are many excellent books out there on diet, so it is not hard to find out what is a healthy diet or a proper diet for diabetes. As we discussed earlier in this chapter, the key principles are:

- Eat a balanced, more plant-based diet.
- Avoid big portions, especially at dinner time.
- Choose foods wisely. Minimize consumption of highly processed foods and carbohydrates like bread, cakes, and cookies.

If you have bad eating habits, remember, they are just habits. You can change your habits. Start by mindfully paying attention to your current eating patterns. In our busy lives processed foods are understandably the go-to choice. But with some planning and effort a new habit can be established and made to fit into our busy lives.

In some ways, one of the most important habits to change is our attitude about food. Food is also medicine for our bodies. When you are establishing your new habit, ask yourself, "Will my body respond well to what I'm about to eat?"

2. Stress Management

Stress can make glucose control extremely difficult. When you are stressed your body thinks you are in danger and makes more sugar available to so that you can either run away or turn and fight with more energy—the flight-or-fight response. If you are a diabetic, you need to manage your stress reaction. We recommend developing a restorative practice that includes meditation along with some sort of meditative movement, such as qigong or taiji. Of course you need to find the technique that is right for you so you can establish a balance in your life between work and relaxation, activity and stillness.

In one of our previous books, *True Wellness: The Mind*, we talked about many of these strategies for stress management, and in chapter 6 of this book, we give you qigong exercises specific for digestive and metabolic health.

3. Physical Activity

Because of overwork, some people feel they don't have time or energy to be physically active. Feeling tired and lethargic can start a vicious cycle. You're tired from work so you don't engage in physical activity. Lack of physical activity contributes to your lack of energy. So you end up feeling even more tired and lethargic, making matters worse.

Physical activity does not mean you need to exercise in the traditional sense. Our ancestors would laugh at us, spending time and money going to the gym when we could be very physically active around our homes and neighborhoods by gardening, cleaning vigorously, and taking long walks with friends. Movement is a mindset and it should be included in our daily lives. Any regular physical activity can be considered exercise. Exercise is not the same as overwork or hard labor. Exercise is "constructive"; overwork is "destructive." Exercise improves and then maintains body function; overwork involves repetitive use of the body and abuses the body. Overwork depletes body energy, but exercise replenishes the body with energy. Over time your body may break down from overuse and you may fall ill.

Your busy life may make you feel like you don't have time for physical activity. As with diet, this is a habit you can change. Once again, mindfully pay attention to your habits. Do you have ten minutes to do a simple but effective qigong exercise? Maybe only five minutes? Good. Take that time. But take that time several times a day. Many recent studies have shown that actively moving for a minimum of twenty-five minutes a day has significant benefits to health and longevity. The so-called Blue Zone areas, where people have the longest life spans, reveal that a lifestyle of moving is a common factor contributing to their healthy longevity. Also monitor the amount of time you spend sitting. Sit for less than 9.5 hours per day.

Our attitudes toward exercise need to change if we are going to change our habits. Simple changes like adding a qigong movement every hour, or just getting up every hour and moving around can contribute greatly to your overall health. Qigong is particularly effective because it was developed to promote beneficial energetic circulation in the body. Look at housework or gardening as an opportunity to move rather than as a chore. Park in the farthest parking space. Climb up stairs rather than take the elevator. But take the elevator to go down. Walking down stairs can be stressful on the joints and can be more dangerous. Move around when you're watching television.

4. Qigong

Qigong has been used for centuries for healing and health, but there are other reasons to develop your practice. If you have diabetes and other GI illnesses, I (Aihan Kuhn) recommend the "Therapeutic Qigong" set. In my practice I have found it to be very effective. This qigong set works on the entire body, opens the channels, improves circulation, and benefits the autonomic nervous system. Qigong promotes better function of all organ systems, and therefore the body's metabolism naturally improves. Even if you still need to use medication to treat your diabetes, you may find that your blood sugar is better controlled on lower doses. Always discuss any medication changes with your healthcare provider prior to making adjustments.

In chapter 6, we discuss the many benefits of qigong in greater detail and you can start your practice with the exercises there.

THE TRUE WELLNESS
APPROACH TO DIABETES

- Adopt a plant-based diet, such as the Mediterranean Diet, that maximizes vegetables and fruit and minimizes simple carbohydrates like breads and pasta
- Move more by doing activities you enjoy. Strive to be active most days of the week
- Decrease stress by using techniques such as meditation, taiji, and qigong
- Follow your doctor's recommendations regarding medications and do not make dose adjustments without their knowledge.
- Consider supplements and botanicals with your doctor's approval:
    - chromium 200–1000 mcg daily
    - alpha-lipoic acid 50–100 mg daily
    - vitamin D 1000–4000 units daily
    - omega 3 fatty acids 1–4 grams daily
    - magnesium 200–500mg/day
    - pycnogenol 100–200 mg daily

CHAPTER 5

The True Wellness Approach to Obesity

I N RECENT YEARS, there has been a lot of finger-pointing going on about who or what is responsible for the obesity epidemic. There are many socioeconomic and biological factors at work. Our food industry produces vast amounts of food-like substances, the ingredients of which are heavily subsidized by taxpayers' money and are laden with excess calories, decreased fiber, and unnatural additives. Because these products are cheap and plentiful, they have taken up a larger proportion of daily intake, leading to weight gain due to increased calories, inflammation, and slower metabolism. In this country there are areas known as "food deserts" where one cannot find much fresh produce, let alone organically-grown produce. Then there is the difficulty of affording the more expensive, higher quality food. Organic farmers do not benefit from the subsidies that large agricultural business receive, so they must price their harvest appropriately so they can stay in business.

Many people, through choice or necessity, eat overly processed foods that contain simple carbohydrates that wreak havoc on their ability to metabolize glucose and also alter their microbiome. This leads to a change in the variety and relative proportions of bacteria in the gut, which leads to increased gastrointestinal inflammation, increased calorie absorption, and increased risk of weight gain and related illnesses. Much depends upon the balance of your microbiome. You may have heard the Cherokee parable of the two wolves that live and battle within each of us. One is evil and the other, good. Which one wins, you ask? The one you feed. Your microbiome works in much the same fashion. If you feed your microbiome lots of vegetables and fruits, you encourage the bacteria that allow many beneficial changes. Your metabolism functions more efficiently, inflammation decreases, and your sense of hunger and satiety normalizes. If you eat excessive amounts of highly processed food-like substances, you will favor the bacteria that encourage weight gain, chronic inflammation, and overeating.

There is some data to suggest that gut bacteria that flourish on sugar can manipulate your enteric nervous system and brain to increase cravings for refined carbohydrates.[1] But there is also evidence that the reverse is true. You can use your brain to influence your behavior and eating habits to cultivate the gut bacteria that contribute to vibrant well-being. In this chapter, we will show you techniques and modalities that will make it easier for you to choose health-promoting foods and activities, allowing your "good" bacteria to flourish.

As you can see, to successfully reverse obesity, you need a multipronged approach. As we discussed in chapter 2, the sudden increase in obesity rates during the last half-century has many underlying causes. The biochemical reactions that dictate the efficiency of your metabolism are dependent upon many factors: your genetics, your microbiome, your sleep patterns, your medications, your environment, and the type and quality of food you eat. It is too simplistic to look only at calorie intake versus calorie output. It is not just a matter of willpower.

Changing how much you weigh may involve more than just changing your eating and exercise habits. This is not just about the body. You have to take the mind and spirit into account and may need to reassess some other aspects of your life. Are you working too hard? Are you sleep-deprived? Are you having relationship problems?

It can be hard to tackle these issues alone. Do you have someone to help you rebalance your life? Your doctor could be that person, guiding you through the whole process. Your physician can address any underlying medical conditions that contribute to, or result from, being overweight. She can also refer you to colleagues such as a nutritionist, an exercise therapist, or a sleep specialist. Often obesity is associated with depression or anxiety. If appropriate, your physician can attend to these problems or

---

1. Joe Alcock, Carlo C. Maley, and C. Athena Aktipis, "Is Eating Behavior Manipulated by the Gastrointestinal Microbiota? Evolutionary Pressures and Potential Mechanisms," *BioEssays* 36. no. 10 (Oct 2014), 940–949.

refer you for counseling. Support groups and health coaches are also very beneficial when undertaking a dramatic lifestyle change.

There are many factors that contribute to obesity, so there may be many changes you need to make to treat it.

Now, let's look at some features of the Western approach to treating obesity.

Diet

We have already written at great length about the importance of a nutrition plan based on abundant vegetables and fruits. Such plans include the Mediterranean Diet and the Anti-Inflammatory Diet. While these regimens were not specifically developed for weight reduction, most people who adopt these eating styles do lose weight. The most important aspect of these diets is their ability to decrease chronic inflammation.

There have been many types of diets that promote weight loss through calorie reduction, but the exact proportions of carbohydrates, protein, and fats differ. Some advocate low carbohydrate/high protein, some recommend eliminating all carbohydrates, and others promote low-fat vegetarianism. The best feature that these regimens have in common is that they focus on eating an abundance of plants. Regardless of the type of eating program, it has been shown that people will lose weight if they consistently follow the plan. Just as the "best" sort of exercise is the one that you will actually do, the "best" diet is the one that you will adopt long term. Over time, your nutritional choices must shift from just being part of a diet to simply being the way you naturally eat.

Provided you are getting adequate amounts of calories, protein, vitamins, and minerals, you can individualize your diet plan according to your own tastes. Diets that advocate extreme calorie restriction are not recommended. Aim for small decreases in your caloric intake through portion control and increasing fruits and vegetables, thereby boosting insoluble fiber content. If you try to cut too many calories, your brain will react as though it is actually starving and will lower your metabolism. This is how strict diets can actually make you fat. Also, such diets are difficult to stick with over the long haul. People tend to gain back even more weight than they lost because their metabolism is slower than when they started dieting. Small changes over a long period of time are your best bet. It may take longer, but your weight loss is more likely to be permanent.

Movement as Medicine

"If exercise could be purchased in a pill, it would be the single most widely prescribed and beneficial medicine in the nation."

—Robert Butler, MD, Former Director of the National Institute on Aging

Exercise is proven to be a very effective component of any weight reduction program. Not only will exercise burn more calories, it will strengthen your heart, lower your blood pressure, and increase your lung function. Exercise will improve your metabolism, your sleep, and your mood. The trick to reaping all these benefits is simply starting to move.

Most of us do not exercise regularly.   In spite of all the gym memberships, workout videos, and athletic gear we purchase, the fact is that only 20 percent of American adults get enough exercise. The national recommendations are that people age eighteen and older get at least thirty minutes of moderate-intensity aerobic exercise or fifteen minutes of vigorous-intensity activity, at least five days per week. Of course, you can divide up your activities as you wish in order to get a combination of both moderate and intense exercise. You could also do more exercise on one day and less on another, as long as the minutes all add up (150 minutes of moderate activity or 75 minutes of vigorous activity). Additionally, you should also do muscle-strengthening activities, like weightlifting, at least twice a week.

If thirty minutes will not fit into your schedule, you may be interested in trying high intensity interval training, known as HIIT. This method can be applied to any form of movement. Research has shown that if you alternate short periods of vigorous activity with low intensity movement in a recovery phase, you will gain the same benefits as if you had exercised moderately for a longer period of time.[2] As little as five to ten minutes a

---

2. Martin J. Gibala, Jonathan P. Little, Maureen J. MacDonal, and John A. Hawley, "Physiological Adaptations to Low-Volume, High-Intensity Interval Training in

day will yield results! You can do this sort of activity anywhere. You do not need to be running on a treadmill or swimming in an Olympic-sized pool. You could be walking up and down your block, dancing in your living room, or doing yard work. All you have to do is perform your chosen activity intensely enough to raise your heart and respiration rate for whatever interval you desire, then continue your activity at a much slower pace to recover for the same amount of time. Your high-intensity interval could be as short as twenty seconds. Ensure that your recovery interval is long enough for your heart rate to lower and your breathing to normalize. This could be anywhere from two to five minutes depending upon your level of fitness. Simply repeat the cycle of high then low intensity movement as many times as you wish to reach your goal for the day.

High intensity interval training is excellent for increasing speed and strength, but your body needs a variety of movement intensities for different reasons. Slower paced cardiovascular exercises like walking, easy swimming, or jogging at a pace that allows conversation are very beneficial. These sorts of exercise allow the body to better utilize fat as fuel and eliminate metabolic by-products. This slower-paced exercise is known as sub-maximal intensity steady-state exercise (SISS) because, just as the name suggests, your effort remains constant and much less than your maximum throughout the time you are moving.

Probably the most important type of interval training is something known as SIIT: sub-maximal intensity interval training. This means the day-to-day activities of living, like walking your dog or vacuuming your floors. We are all spending more and more time sitting, whether for work or leisure. If this increase in sitting time encroaches on our activity time, serious health conditions can result.[3] You may have heard the saying that "sitting is the new smoking," implying that sitting will harm you just as smoking cigarettes can. What seems to be closer to the truth is that the lack of regular movement over the course of your day will increase your risk of disease and death.

Health and Disease," *The Journal of Physiology* 590, no. 5: 1077–1084, https://doi. org/10.1113/jphysiol.2011.224725

3. I. M. Lee, E. J. Shiroma, f. Lobelo et al., "Effect of Physical Inactivity on Major Non-Communicable Diseases Worldwide: An Analysis of Burden of Disease and Life Expectancy," *Lancet* 380 (9838):219–229.

In fact, there was a very large, prospective long-term study performed by the American Cancer Society that followed 123,000 middle-aged adults over fourteen years that demonstrated that lack of movement increased the risk of dying. The researchers found that women who sat the most were 34 percent more likely to die from *any* cause than women who sat the least. For men, the likelihood was 17 percent. If exercise was taken into consideration the difference was staggering. The women who were most sedentary, meaning they did not do regular exercise or move a lot in their day-to-day activities, were approximately twice as likely to die from any cause than those who both exercised and moved the most. Looking at the same categories for the men, the risk for the most sedentary was 50 percent.[4] An interesting point to note is that exercise alone did not confer the most benefit. Even if you work out for 150 minutes per week, you are at greater risk of dying earlier if you sit around and do nothing else in your daily life. The longest-lived people on the planet are those that incorporate natural, low-intensity movement as part of their normal day. Dan Buettner chronicled this finding when he went around the world and looked at lifestyles of healthy centenarians in various societies from the Okinawans to the Sardinians, halfway around the world.[5]

We realize that we cannot all be Sardinian shepherds who walk miles in the course of a day. There is no escaping the fact that a lot of us earn our living working in front of computers, but we need to counter the lack of activity by purposefully adding movement back into our lives. Therefore, throughout the day, get up and move for two to five minutes for every hour that you are sitting. You could walk around your office building or climb a flight of stairs. Qigong exercises are an excellent choice to get your blood flowing, relieve muscle tension, and alleviate stress.

It is important to have diversity in the intensity of your interval training. You may not feel up to any sort of high intensity movement at all. Not everyone is an athlete and for the 80 percent of us who do not exercise regularly, even five minutes a day can be daunting. The best way to start

---

4. A. V. Patel et al, "Leisure Time Spent Sitting in Relation to Total Mortality in a Prospective Cohort of US Adults," *American Journal of Epidemiology* 172, no. 4 (Aug. 15 2010): 419–429, https://doi.org/ 10.1093/aje/kwql55.

5. Dan Buettner, "The Blue Zones: Lessons for Living Longer from the People Who've Lived the Longest,"(Washington, DC: *National Geographic*, 2008), 223.

exercising is simply to start moving. It doesn't matter what you do—walking, dancing, gardening, cleaning, hiking, skateboarding, swimming, whatever you enjoy. This sort of activity has been dubbed non-exercise activity thermogenesis (NEAT)[6] as it does burn about 350 calories per day. At the beginning, it also does not matter how many minutes you are active, so long as you do *something* regularly. Planning an activity with a friend or relative will increase the likelihood that you will meet your goal. We are more willing to disappoint ourselves than another person. You can use this foible of human nature to launch your regular movement routine. Do not forget to reward yourself for your efforts. As we mentioned earlier, we establish habits more easily if our efforts are rewarded. Once you start to move, you will feel better on so many different levels and you will want to continue. After several weeks, you will have established the habit of regular movement. At this point, you can start to increase the duration and intensity of your chosen activity, remembering that hourly, short-duration, low-intensity movement is your best bet to establish the habit of movement and achieve optimal health.

Stress Management

Stress can contribute to obesity. As we have explained previously, when you are under stress, your body releases various hormones, including cortisol. Chronically elevated cortisol levels are associated with abdominal obesity as well as other physiological derangements. When you are stressed, your nervous system is out of balance. Techniques that bring equilibrium to your sympathetic and parasympathetic nervous systems include meditation, taiji, and qigong. These therapies, along with hypnosis and biofeedback, can decrease stress, lower cortisol levels, decrease inflammation, create a sense of calm, and lead to better choices around food. In the segment on Eastern approaches to obesity, various options to relieve stress will be discussed.

---

6. J. A. Levine, "Nonexercise Activity Thermogenesis—Liberating the Life-force," *Journal of Internal Medicine* 262, no. 3 (Sept. 2007): 273–287.

Health Coaching

Some people think, "Why on earth would I need someone to help me lose weight? All I have to do is just say no to the foods that are making me fat and get out and exercise more." Well, if it were that simple, no one would be obese. Aside from the environmental, genetic, and socioeconomic factors we discussed, many people have to contend with the low self-esteem that results when they are unable to stick with the plan they have created for weight loss. They feel that they lack self-control or are lazy. Self-loathing and depression can follow. The body perceives these emotions as stressors and is driven to find ways to calm the fight-or-flight response. One very common way of soothing these emotions is through eating. A vicious cycle ensues, and a health coach can help break that cycle.

Unfortunately, the self-control paradigm does not work for most people. Studies have shown that those who really can "just say no" are intrinsically less interested in behaviors that should be avoided (e.g., eating the donut) and more interested in performing positive behaviors like being more active. Moreover, people who feel that they are good at avoiding temptation and are better at self-control have developed habits that make healthy choices automatic.[7] A health coach can help you create these habits by examining the current situation with you in a realistic fashion, then helping you decide what it is you really want to achieve. Then, they can help you break down these goals into virtually effortless actions. If something is ridiculously easy and also enjoyable, the likelihood of you taking action is increased. Over time, these small steps build into habits. These habits yield positive outcomes and reinforce the healthy behavior.

More Aggressive Medical Interventions

Using drugs or surgery to lose weight has become very common in America and, for some people, these modalities are their last hope. If you are entertaining these options you need to clearly understand their risks, ben-

---

7. Brian M. Galla and Angela L. Duckworth, "More than Resisting Temptation: Beneficial Habits Mediate the Relationship between Self-Control and Positive Life Outcomes," *Journal of Personality and Social Psychology* 109, no. 3 (Sept. 2015): 508–525, https://doi.org/10.1037/pspp0000026.

efits, and alternatives. Weight-loss drugs and surgery are not recommended for everyone and we do not advocate their use before a concerted effort is made by a patient with as much support from both Western and Eastern practitioners as can be mustered. Regular visits with a dietician to improve food choices and health coaching are even paid for by some health insurances companies. Many have set up their own weight-loss programs that have the additional benefit of community support. Acupuncture is excellent to decrease stress and improve mood, leading to better decisions around food selection and motivation to engage in physical activity. Meditation is very calming and increases focus. Referral to a psychologist can also be helpful in healing from the various traumas that can lead to overeating. All these modalities have a part to play in weight loss and should be thoroughly investigated before considering drugs or surgery.

If such drugs or surgery are necessary, they should only be prescribed or performed by doctors who have subspecialized in the field of weight loss. This new subspecialty is called "bariatric medicine." The word "bariatric" is derived from the Greek word "bar," meaning "weight." The goal of doctors who specialize in bariatric medicine is to control and treat obesity and its associated diseases.

Referral to a specialist in bariatric medicine could be considered for any patient who has been unable to lose weight after genuinely trying for more than six months and has a BMI of thirty or higher. Some doctors might refer their patients at a BMI of twenty-seven if they have a comorbid condition like diabetes or high blood pressure.

There are two types of prescription drugs that are used for weight loss. The first type works as an appetite suppressant and also increases metabolism (phentermine, brand name Adipex-PTM). This medication has a chemical structure similar to amphetamine. The possible side effects include insomnia, palpitations, high blood pressure, dry mouth, constipation, seizures (though rarely), and lung or heart problems. The second type stops fat absorption from your intestines (orlistat, brand name—Xenical™). The main side effects of this drug results from its mechanism of action. Because the fat in the food you eat is not absorbed well, your stools become oily. This can cause abdominal pain, loss of control of your bowels, and gas. The manufacturer recommends that you eat low-fat, calorie-reduced meals to avoid these side effects. One would think that if you followed these recommendations, you would lose weight anyway.

All that said, people have lost weight using these medications. If you decide to try either type of diet drug you should be supervised by a physician. The length of time that you could stay on these drugs varies. You can still regain the weight you lost if you do not change your eating habits.

For those people who have not been able to lose any weight with lifestyle changes and medications, there remains the option of surgery. This method could be considered in a patient whose BMI is forty or higher (or thirty-five and higher with medical comorbidities). Candidates for surgical interventions must also have tried to lose weight under medical supervision for at least six months.

The types of surgery most commonly used include adjustable gastric banding and gastric bypass. Gastric banding will reduce your stomach volume and is classified as a "restrictive" procedure. Gastric bypass not only restricts stomach size but also bypasses a considerable part of your duodenum, the part of your small intestine that will absorb food. This procure is classified as a "combined restrictive and malabsorptive" procedure.

These surgical procedures can produce significant weight loss and reverse hypertension and type-2 diabetes. However, they are not without risk. Surgical complications can result in up to 10 percent of cases and death can occur in about three in one thousand procedures. If you are referred for consideration of a surgical technique you will undergo an extensive preoperative workup including physical exam, laboratory tests, and psychological evaluation.

Even with these aggressive medical and surgical interventions it is imperative that you change your eating habits. It is possible to "override" the above treatments and still gain weight while on medications or after surgery. Given the possibility of complications with such interventions, up to and including death, we feel that modifying your behavior and lifestyle is still the safest way to improve your health. We have seen our patients make these changes gradually and successfully, supported by the modalities of Eastern medicine.

Eastern Approach to Healing Obesity

In Eastern healing, we see the digestive system as one of the most important organ systems. The digestive system affects the whole body, including energy and emotions. If the digestive system is not functioning well, sooner or later other organ systems may suffer. In treating obesity, when the digestive function is out of balance, not only is the obesity difficult to treat, but the person very likely has other medical issues, such as high cholesterol, diabetes, cardiovascular or respiratory problems, liver or gall bladder issues, other metabolic problems, or even cancer.

In Chinese medicine, the "Spleen" is one of the primary organ systems involved in digestion, absorption, and elimination. The "Spleen" we are discussing here is not the Spleen you think of in Western anatomical terms. Rather, it is an energetic and functional system. When doctors who practice Eastern medicine see a patient with digestive concerns, they often say "Pi Wei" are not good, which means the Spleen and Stomach systems are not functioning well. The Spleen governs movement and transformation, while the Stomach governs intake. The formation of "qi" (vital energy), blood, and body fluids relies on the Spleen-Stomach function of moving and transforming the essence of food and water. This pair is the root of the acquired constitution, which is another way of describing a person's state of health. The Small and Large Intestines are connected by channels to the Heart and the Lung. You may recall in your own experience, your breathing would be shallow and your energy would be low when you either eat too much or too little.

In addition to ingestion and transforming, the Spleen manages the blood and it is the source of qi and blood formation. Because of this, the Spleen also governs the muscles in the limbs. When someone is overweight or underweight, their muscles tend to be weak. Furthermore, the Spleen is related to the taste of the mouth. If you don't have an appetite, can't taste your food, or have bad breath, you know you have a problem with your Spleen.

The Liver and Kidney systems can also affect the Spleen. The Liver is associated with mood and emotion in addition to other functions. If you feel depressed, you may also experience an eating or drinking disorder, or some digestive problems. Similarly, if you are lacking in Kidney qi, especially Kidney yang (Kidney has yin energy and yang energy), you may have poor digestion and absorption.

Some causes for Spleen energy imbalance may be associated with a poor diet that might include fried foods, sweets, refined foods, and an overconsumption of raw foods and iced drinks. Overthinking and worrying can also affect Spleen energy. Often, digestive problems related to Spleen qi deficiency will have elements of Dampness. Dampness is an interesting concept in Eastern medicine. The symptoms of Dampness include sticky stools, a distended abdomen, abdominal pain, and weight problems. If a person has Spleen Dampness, they may experience a bloated sensation or the feeling of body swelling or puffiness.

Maintaining healthy digestive energy is especially important for women. Keeping healthy stomach function helps to prevent breast cancer, too. In Eastern medicine, the stomach channels go through the breasts. If the Stomach channel is blocked, it affects energy flow of the breasts. By investigating a breast cancer patient's medical history, excluding genetic factors, I (Dr. Kuhn) have found that many of them in their lifetime had some kind of problem with their digestive function. Certainly, obesity increases the risk for breast cancer.[8]

Preserving stomach energy is a big part of preserving one's daily energy level too. Just recall your daily life: What do you feel after eating a big lunch or dinner? What do you feel after eating huge holiday dinners? We have so many parties in November, December, and early January, even February. We end up feeling bloated and tired, and we need a solution. Every January, many people make a New Year's resolution to lose weight and sign up at a gym. But, as many have discovered, this resolution is not easy to keep.

Eating when stressed or feeling emotional is another issue that affects the energetic systems. These are the most dangerous diet habits and contribute to many illnesses. Without learning to manage stress and balance emotion, weight loss is not easy.

Overeating is very common. Fueled by stress and our fast-paced lifestyles, we rush through our meals. Most of us are not aware of what we're

---

8. Centers for Disease Control and Prevention, "What Are the Risk Factors for Breast Cancer?" https://www.cdc.gov/cancer/breast/basic_info/risk_factors.htm.

eating. We don't take time to taste food, chew food, feel the food, and connect food with our body.

Added to that, eating the wrong food is very common in our modern world. The commercial food industry does not help either. So many of the foods we are drawn to, partly because they are convenient, have preservatives and ingredients harmful to our systems.

To solve these problem takes a multilayered approach. We need to ask ourselves: "What do I want for my health?" "What do I have to do to get what I want?" "How do I manage my life to do what is necessary to reach my goals?" When your mind is clear, your healing path becomes easier. The next step is action.

Maintaining Optimum Weight Naturally

For many people, losing weight is not hard, but maintaining the optimum weight is extremely difficult. In attempts to lose weight, some people go to dietary specialists, buy books on each new diet fad, join weight loss organizations, take diet pills, or undergo surgery; and some even starve themselves. Some people develop complications after trying some of these approaches and often regain the weight.

In weight control, in addition to diet and physical activity, management of stress is crucial. People who are stressed tend to eat poorly and exercise less, which exacerbates weight problems and associated health issues. We will discuss more about this shortly.

Obtaining and maintaining a healthy weight involves multiple approaches. In Eastern medicine we incorporate healing treatments such as acupuncture and tui na (Chinese bodywork), dietary therapy, daily exercise, qigong, a positive mindset, and Daoist wisdom.

Intention

Training your mind to strengthen your intention, your belief in yourself, and your determination are key factors to effective weight loss and maintenance. A positive outlook is a habit that can be developed. You have to be ready in order to achieve your optimum weight and health. Take the time to gather information related to your health and weight. Once you are ready, you can start your weight loss journey. When your mind is determined and your intention is clear, you are more prepared to accomplish your goals.

First, you have to believe in yourself. Your belief helps to create positive energy that directs your action toward the goal. Then your determination and persistence really lead you there. Practice mindfulness daily. The practice trains your mind to stay focused on your daily actions and this awareness helps you stay on your path. Engaging in practices like qigong, taiji, or yoga also help you develop mindful awareness. This attitude is one of the keys to success.

Your thoughts hold great power. This is not simply magical thinking. The science of epigenetics has revealed how your thoughts influence your gene expression and therefore how your body functions. For a long time we thought that gene expression could not change, that your genes were your destiny. The scientific opinion was that overweight bodies could not change. But scientists have discovered how our genes are turned off or turned on can be changed by what you eat, how you move, and what you think. This is how you can heal your body.

I recommend Dr. Catherine Shanahan's book "Deep Nutrition." She clearly describes the science of epigenetics. In her book, she made this statement: "Whether you believe in the idea of genetic intelligence or not, the one thing I hope I have made clear in this chapter is that our genes are not written in stone. They are exquisitely sensitive to how we treat them."

Our mind plays a big part roll in weight loss. Practice thinking differently about food and diet. Your thoughts can influence your actions. Think of messages that help you stay on track. Use your own name before each thought. Saying your own name out loud gets your brain's attention. Use this tool to help you make good food decisions. Here are a few suggestions.

> "Aihan, you know this food is tasty, but you know it is not healthy. Think of how you will feel if you eat it."
>
> "Catherine, think about your health, not just about pleasing your mouth."
>
> "Aihan, eating late is not good for your health. Have this treat tomorrow."
>
> "Catherine, think about your health. You can make the right choice."

I had a patient who came to me for help with her weight problem. It was the end of May, and she wanted to be thin in the summer so she could wear a bathing suit at the beach and look good. But while she was on vacation, she would not give up the enjoyment of food. For her, summer vacation was not a time for discipline in her diet. She was clearly not ready to make a change, so I suggested she start her weight loss program in the fall when she is truly ready. The point is that you have to know what you really want and when you are ready.

Eight Steps to Successful Weight Loss

1. Keep a Positive Attitude. Losing weight and maintaining a healthy weight is a journey. In this journey your mind is most important in the journey, Not only do you have to be determined to lose weight but you also have to be positive during the process. Sometimes you don't see results as quickly as you expected, but don't lose faith or give up. Be patient: losing weight takes time. Taking small steps and developing a new habit of eating and a new attitude toward food will contribute to long-term success. Taking small steps can help make the transition smooth and steady. During the process, try to listen to yourself and know what you really want, know what works, what doesn't work, and how you feel.

When you are about lose your discipline, think about your goal, your journey, and your healing.

2. Build a Healthy Shopping List. Before you go shopping for groceries, make a list. Think about nutritious, chemical-free, organic, plant-based, quality foods.

To avoid making impulse purchases that may not be very healthy and buying more than you need, try not to go to the market when you are hungry.

What is good food and what is bad food? This can be a very confusing question. Some foods that are good for certain people may not be good for others. In most cases you can figure out what foods are good or not good for you by paying attention to how the food makes you feel. If what you eat makes you uncomfortable, causes indigestion, makes you feel bloated, causes you to gain weight, you will need to modify your diet.

In general, focus on plant-based foods:
- green leafy vegetables and other colored vegetables
- fruits
- whole grains
- sorghum, millet, rye, barley
- quinoa
- nuts and seeds
- avocados
- berries
- beans or bean products
- plants that grow in the ocean, such as seaweed
- fermented foods
- dark chocolate

Foods you should avoid:
- foods high in fat, especially saturated fat
- foods high in sugar, except fruits (fruits have natural sugar and reasonable amounts of it)
- simple carbohydrates (bleached flour products such as white bread, pasta, rice, cookies, cakes, and muffins)
- red meat
- dairy
- fried foods
- foods that contain preservatives, food coloring, and other additives
- salt in excess

Be in tune with your body and your mind. Listen to your body. Your body is trying to tell you what is beneficial and what is not. For instance, some people experience headaches after eating chocolate, some people feel bloated after eating cheese, and others feel tired after eating a lot of grains. These symptoms are your body telling you it dislikes such foods.

Occasionally we all eat unhealthy foods, and that is ok. For instance, around the holidays we often eat foods that contain high calories and sugar. But after the holidays, help your body recover by eating healthily again. If you know an event is coming up where there will lots of delicious but maybe not so nutritious treats available, prepare your body by making sure you eat healthful foods before the event. You may even find that you are less tempted as your body adjusts to a healthy diet. Sugar in particular is a highly addictive substance and when we limit the sugar in our diets, our cravings lessen. Progress in your journey to health step by step.

3. Learn Healthy Cooking. If you don't know how to cook, or even if you already do, you can find inspiration and instruction from the many cookbooks available on healthy cooking. There are countless cookbooks covering all kinds of cuisines. When it comes to information we are fortunate to live in a cyberworld, and we can easily get information from the Internet including healthy cooking recipes. Many of them are quick and easy. Take a class and share recipes with friends. You will find that eating healthfully is not torture but a tasty journey with many paths.

Cooking various types of food has the added benefit of being a brain exercise. The preparation for cooking—choosing what to make, what spices to use, and how to put different foods together into a satisfying meal—call upon various activities in the brain. This is also a mindfulness practice that stimulates and activates our brain. If you don't know how to cook, follow a recipe. The more you cook, the better cook you will become. Learning healthy cooking is also good for our emotions. Not only is the brain activated, the flavors also help boost neurotransmitters in the brain that improve mood. These neurotransmitters include dopamine, oxytocin, endorphins, serotonin, and endocannabinoids.[9]

4. Quantity. Have you noticed that we eat too much food, especially at dinnertime? This is linked to our lifestyle: we don't have much time in the morning and noon, so we have to have a large meal at dinner. We have already talked about how eating in accordance with our natural circadian rhythm is more healthful, specifically by finishing our last meal of the day by about 7 p.m.—a tricky feat in this day and age. But, have you heard an expression, "Where there's a will, there's a way"? There is always a way to do what's important, including develop healthy eating habits. Habit is the key to improving diets. Though changing habits is sometimes easier said than done, the key is an ongoing mindfulness practice.

The quantity of food we eat can vary between individuals. If you do a lot of physical work or if your body metabolism is high, you need to eat more food and calories. However, most occupations in this cyber world

---

9. Michael Greger, MD, *How Not to Diet* (New York: Flatiron Books, 2019), 174.

involve sitting, which requires much less physical work. Therefore, we need to eat less quantity of food unless we have the discipline to exercise regularly. Otherwise any excess food in our body can cause weight problems, high cholesterol, obesity, and other health problems.

When it is functioning properly, our body tells us to stop eating. We will get this message when we are attuned to our body and mind. But those who are not paying attention or whose gut-brain-microbiome access is impaired may keep eating until they feel stuffed or over bloated. This can lead to more digestive and weight problems.

You can do a self-examination to find out if you have an imbalance in your digestive system: put pressure on the stomach after eating; if you have pain or discomfort over the stomach area, your digestive system has some issues.

5. Build Better Eating Habits: Four-A Practice

First "A": Avoid "Emotional Eating" and "Stress Eating." If we always use foods to deal with our stress, there is imbalance in our energy pathway that affects our organs and brain. Our brain has an emotion center that is located in the limbic system, just under the cerebrum. The limbic system is a complex system that includes the hypothalamus, hippocampus, amygdala, olfactory bulb, and other related areas. The limbic system supports various functions including emotions, behavior, motivation, long-term memory, and eating. When we lose body equilibrium or have an organ imbalance, our limbic system has lost its self-regulating function and causes us to "do as we wish," but not in a logical way. We do not think rationally and ask, "Is this right or not"?

Eating when we are emotional or stressed is very common, especially in women. This happens because your body is reacting to a stressful situation, and sugary comfort foods actually decrease the cortisol levels in your brain and release neurotransmitters that elevate your mood. This impacts the limbic system. Emotional eating is a way to overcome a crisis. But afterward you may want to think whether this is really the right method for stress reduction. Is there another way to deal with your stress? When you question yourself, you will most likely find that better way. This is a mindfulness practice.

If you always use food to relieve your stress, you may end up seeing more doctors more often for more health problems. You may also have a hard time losing weight.

The first thing is to recognize emotional eating when it happens and try to stop the behavior right then. Find out why you are emotional or what is causing your stress, and use other methods to develop healthier habits.

Here are some ideas and suggestions you can do to help yourself:
- Get out of the house and go for a walk or a bike ride. The fresh air will help make you feel better. If you can't go outside, walk around the house a few times or put on music and dance.
- Eat a healthy snack if you have to eat: carrots, celery, apples, nuts, and seeds, but nothing in large portions.
- Watch a movie with friends, or watch a comedy show.
- Clean your house or room. Organize your work or your office. This can redirect your mind and give you a little break from overthinking.
- Take a bath while listening to relaxing music.
- Call friends or family just to chat, no need to make any point.
- Practice qigong exercises (chapter 6 of this book).
- Learn and practice qigong or taiji to help you manage stress better.
- Practice daily meditation to relieve stress; even just five minutes can be effective.

If you think you have an addiction, you should seek help from either Western or Eastern methods. Both can help you to overcome the addiction. And don't hesitate to seek professional help to untangle the underlying reasons you are eating to relieve stress. You may want to speak to a counselor about some of these issues rather than a friend or family member. Acupuncture is also a great healing modality to decrease stress levels, balance neurotransmitters, and elevate endorphins.

Second "A": Avoid Eating Late. Eating late contributes to weight problems and diseases such as heart disease, hypertension, high cholesterol, and diabetes. It also exacerbates respiratory illness, digestive issues, and other conditions. We explained in chapter 2, in the section "How the Sleep-Wake Cycle Affects the Gut," why this can happen. From the Eastern medical point of view, the energy at night is not optimal for the digestive system.

Many people eat late because of work and commuting schedules. There is probably nothing wrong with this if you are able to keep active for at least three hours after eating and if you don't go to bed immediately after eating. What I mean by "active" is doing some walking, housework, qigong, taiji, or stretching. Then you can relax with a book or the TV. It does not mean you have to lift weights or go running several miles. Moving assists your stomach and intestines digest your food and absorb its nutrients.

Try not to have a big meal when you come home late. A light dinner can be still very delicious. Have easily digested foods like a vegetable stir-fry, salad, soup, nuts, or seeds. Eating a huge meal just before bedtime often has an adverse effect on restful sleep. Many people who have insomnia may also have poor eating habits.

Third "A": Avoid Getting Too Hungry. We often eat more than normal when we are hungry. When we are hungry, we eat faster than normal, and our brain does not have enough time to recognize that we are actually full. We keep eating and eating and by the time our brain realizes we are full, we are completely stuffed and it is too late. To avoid this, eating a healthy snack between meals is good habit to develop. It can prevent hunger and overeating. Another habit you can cultivate is taking time to chew your food.

If you are too hungry before going to bed, low blood sugar could adversely affect your sleep, which is not good either. High blood sugar can also interfere with getting a restful sleep. Therefore, before going to bed, be neither over hungry nor over full. A convenient source of dense nutrition is nuts. If you are NOT allergic to nuts, keep them around for a quick snack. But don't forget, even nuts can harm your digestive system if you eat too many of them. By eating a little about one hour before your next meal, you can avoid being over hungry. If you find that you are hungry before going to bed, consider whether the problem really is that you are staying up too late at night. Allow yourself an eight-hour window for sleep so that you will get at least seven hours of sleep.

Fourth "A": Avoid Soft Drinks. Most soft drinks contain a lot of sugar. In general, we consume much more sugar than we need. There's sugar in coffee, in pastries, in meals themselves, in bread, in snacks. On top of this, we get even more sugar from soft drinks. Increased rates of diabetes are partially due to excess sugar consumption. Nearly thirty-four million Americans have diabetes, according to new estimates from the Centers for

Disease Control and Prevention (CDC). In addition, an estimated eighty-eight million U.S. adults have prediabetes, a condition in which blood sugar levels are higher than normal but not high enough to be diagnosed as diabetes. Prediabetes raises a person's risk of type-2 diabetes, heart disease, and stroke.

6. Create a Healthy Environment. Create a supportive environment for your journey. Fill your pantry and refrigerator with healthy foods. Precut veggies so they are a convenient go-to snack. Ask your friends to join you for a weight loss challenge, or ask your spouse to join you or support you. This can make your work a lot easier. You and your friends can help each other by sharing information and supporting each other to achieve your goals. You could try an organized weight loss program or take an exercise, qigong, or yoga class.

"A goal without a plan is just a wish."

—Antoine de Saint-Exupery

7. Making a Plan. Goal-setting is beneficial in many endeavors: succeeding at school, running a business, leading a company, teaching, financial planning, and achieving optimal health. Take the time to be aware of want you want to achieve, what is important to you, what you need to improve, and what kind of life you want to have. Weight loss is just a step to a greater goal of achieving overall health. The right use of food is just one of the ways you get there. The more healthfully you eat the more healthful you will be.

After you have your bigger goal in place, set smaller goals or steps. Change your diet, exercise more, and remove junk food and sweets. Do therapeutic exercise daily, eat the right foods, take herbs to assist in healing. Change your daily routine, change eating habits, and change lifestyle. All these require mindful practice and determination, but once the new routine is established, it becomes almost effortless.

Everyone's individual plan for achieving optimal health will be different. We all have a different reason for healing or for losing weight, whether it's a chronic physical issue, an emotional issue, or even a desire to have a better relationship with someone.

Many people have a goal in mind but have trouble taking action to achieve that goal. The changes they expect themselves to make are simply too large to be sustainable. Taking small steps toward a larger goal is the key. In her superb book *The Four-Day Win*, Martha Beck likens small changes to the adjustments that are made while navigating a sailboat. The sail settings are fine-tuned to keep the boat on course. It may seem as though a tiny variation will not make a difference, but over time and distance, the effect is significant. Similarly, making one small rewarded adjustment after another creates lasting change in our lives. Beck puts forward a transtheoretical model of change, which explains how people prepare for and implement lifestyle changes over time. While her book is primarily about weight loss, she dovetails the transtheoretical model of change with the Daoist philosophy of moderation and compassion to prepare the reader to achieve their goal.[10]

In the following section we will ask you many questions. Take your time and answer these questions truthfully. These responses will create the scaffolding of your healing plan. Let's get started.

What is your goal?

Try to be specific and set a realistic goal; for example, to lose five pounds.

What are the steps you need to follow to reach your goal?

This is one of the most important parts of creating your plan. There is a lot of information you need to know in order to develop a realistic plan that will yield results. If you want to get your weight under control, you need to make an honest assessment of your current habits. What foods do you eat now? Which contain refined sugars, and what foods would be better substitutes? Can you think of ways to resist the temptation to eat foods that will excessively elevate your sugars? How do you politely decline well-meaning people who insist you try their dessert? What sort of activities do you like? What intensity of exercise are you currently capable of performing without injuring yourself? When and where are you going to engage in these activities and with whom?

---

10. Martha Beck, PhD, *The Four-Day Win: End Your Diet War and Achieve Thinner Peace* (New York: Rodale, 2007), 145.

Breaking down each step like this may seem daunting, but it will give you a lot of insight into how you make changes in your life and why you may not have succeeded in the past.

Write down the steps you are going to follow, making sure that the steps are practical; otherwise, they will be more difficult to accomplish. Do not be ashamed to write down what you may consider to be a ridiculously small change in your habits. As Martha Beck points out, it is the stacking of a series of tiny adjustments that will take you where you want to be. The title of the book, *The Four-Day Win*, refers to the number of days she recommends spending on implementing a change before making another alteration. For each day, you should give yourself a small reward and a slightly larger reward on the fourth day. In her book, she describes how she became an avid exerciser. Her first four-day win consisted of driving to the gym and sitting in the parking lot for three minutes for four consecutive days. Yes, she did reward herself. For the next four days, she went into the gym and pedaled on a stationary bike for three minutes. Over a period of about three weeks, she came to enjoy and benefit from longer and more vigorous exercise sessions.

This is exactly how you should be approaching your goal. Baby steps, consistently applied, will get you much further than an all-out sprint you cannot sustain.

What are the obstacles you faced in the past? Many people failed because they have obstacles they don't recognize or are not able to overcome. Obstacles can be work or living situations, time constraints, and even friends and relatives. Once you know your obstacles, you can mindfully rise above them.

How will you overcome these obstacles?

Sometimes this is the most difficult part, especially if your obstacles are people you love. You have to be creative and find solutions. Whatever the obstacle, there is usually a solution. No time to exercise because you have kids? Take them walking with you, ask a friend or relative to babysit on a regular basis, or trade childcare with another parent.

Consider substituting an enjoyable activity for an unhealthy one. For example, if you are handy, use that skill to supplant a bad habit. Knit, paint, or make jewelry instead of eating to pass the time. Take up woodworking, learn an instrument, go Latin dancing—anything you have always wanted to try.

How will you organize and document your healing plan?

These days there are innumerable electronic and paper organizing systems. You may think these are a waste of time, but people who write down their goals and document their efforts have a greater chance of reaching their target. Choose which system works best for you, but be diligent and use it daily.

It doesn't have to be a fancy device either. For example, most people have a calendar hanging on the wall. All you need to do is to put healing hours on the calendar for each day. Regardless of what kind of work you do or how busy you are, you can make anything happen if you have written information on the calendar and read it daily. You can put down what you're going to eat that day, daily exercise hours, or anything else important that you have to do.

Many of these systems use a worksheet format. It will allow you to write down all the small steps you need to take to reach your goal, giving you a roadmap to follow. You can include your daily physical goals, and you can set mental or emotional goals.

In many industries, checklists improve safety and efficiency. Checklists get results. Checklists also capitalize on the sense of satisfaction we get from crossing off something on our to-do list. Biochemically, this is a little rush of dopamine that rewards you for performing a desired behavior. This is how you develop healthful habits. To that end, we have supplied you with a template for your *True Wellness* checklist that you can modify to suit your dietary preferences.

Another way people succeed in losing weight is to write down everything they eat. And I mean absolutely everything! This brings things into sharp focus. It has been shown that people who keep food journals like this tend to lose more weight and keep it off because they are more mindful of exactly what they are eating.

As for what to eat, your weight loss plan must be tailored to you. No matter whether you choose a Mediterranean diet, veganism, Paleo, or Peganism, the important thing is to make plants the centerpiece of your plan. There are many excellent books and websites outlining each of these approaches and they usually include delicious recipes. Take the time to try each style and then pick the one you enjoy the most because you are most likely to stick with it for life.

Regarding nutrient proportions, these can vary since everyone is different. For instance, if your occupation involves more physical work, your protein portion can be more than for an office worker.

Vegetable and fruits—and be sure to eat a wide variety of them—should be about 50 percent, protein from various sources should be about 20 percent, carbohydrates from grains or resistant starches can be about 25 to 30 percent, and miscellaneous food such as condiments, nuts, seeds, and fats should be about 5 percent.

Now that you have considered the small steps you need to string together to improve your health, document your plan and stick to it as closely as possible. No one is able to implement lifestyle changes perfectly. Use the 80/20 rule. If you are able to follow your plan 80 percent of the time, you will achieve your goal.

8. Qigong Daily. Qigong is a mind-body exercise that is good for your total well-being. We are big fans of qigong because we have received so many health benefits from practicing it. In the next chapter, there is a more in-depth discussion of qigong and a qigong form that is beneficial for weight loss and digestive health.

CHAPTER 6

Qigong to Heal the Gut

THE TERM *QIGONG* is composed of two words. The first, "qi," has been translated as the "life energy" or "vital force" within the body. "Gong" has been translated as "work" or "mastery." Together, the word qigong can be interpreted as "energy work" or the act of mastering one's vital force. Qigong is a healing practice that combines breath control with mental concentration. There are many forms of qigong, but they all basically fall within two types: passive or active. Passive qigong is performed seated or lying down and resembles the postures we associate with meditation. This is also known as internal qigong or nei gong. In the active form of qigong, breath control and focused attention are combined with specific movements to create a type of moving meditation. Active qigong, also known as external qigong or wei gong, is similar to taiji and yoga.

The practice of qigong is an ancient one. These exercises were known by several names over the centuries, including Dao-Yin or "leading and guiding the energy."[1] Earlier in this book we discussed the silk scrolls that were discovered in the Mawangdui tombs in 1973. These silk texts date back to 168 BCE. A chart was found amongst these scrolls that depicted the Dao-Yin postures. The Dao-Yin Tu (Dao-Yin Illustrations) consisted of four rows of eleven postures. In these illustrations, the roots of most modern qigong practices can be found. There were also descriptions of the stances, instructions for the movements, and indications for the use of each exercise. Certain Dao-Yin exercises were deemed valuable in treating low back pain and painful knees, others were indicated for gastrointestinal disorders, and still others were designated to treat anxiety. This demonstrates that not only were Dao-Yin exercises prescribed as a medical

---

1. Kenneth S. Cohen, *The Way of Qigong: The Art and Science of Chinese Energy Healing* (New York: Ballantine Books, 1997), 13.

therapy, but that ancient physicians appreciated the utility of this type of qigong practice in the treatment of emotional disharmony.[2]

As old as qigong is, its development was likely influenced by the older Indian practice of yoga. The earliest known documentation of yoga was found in the Indus Valley and dates back five thousand years. Millennia later, in approximately 1000 BCE, the Upanishads were written. These commentaries emphasize the personal, experiential nature of the journey toward spirituality and elucidate many basic yoga teachings, promoting an understanding of the principles of karma, chakras, meditation, and prana.[3] In India, the vital life force is known as "prana," and pranayama is the cultivation of the life force through breath control. By breathing with intention, the prana is moved through the nadi (channels). The intersections of important nadi are called chakras. There are many similarities between this system of energy management and that of qigong and Eastern medicine. Qigong requires the same attention to and control of the breath and movement of qi through channels of the body. Interestingly, the locations of many important acupuncture points correspond to the positions of the chakras.

While yoga and taiji have many benefits, we feel that qigong is the best practice if you are new to these Eastern healing arts, especially if you have any physical limitations that prevent prolonged standing or impede your ability to move between standing and lying positions. Whether you practice nei gong or wei gong, the regulation of the following components are related and inseparable: the body, the breath, the mind (thoughts), the qi, and the spirit (emotions).[4] The purpose of regulating and strengthening these components is to achieve good health and longevity.

These related and inseparable elements can also be understood, in a traditional sense, as the "Three Treasures"—*jing, qi,* and *shen.* In Eastern medicine, the Three Treasures are considered the root of life. The *jing* is often translated as essence and, in a Western sense, is akin to your genetic

2. Cohen, *Way of Qi Gong,* 13.

3. Jennie Lee, *True Yoga: Practicing with the Yoga Sutras for Happiness and Spiritual Fulfillment* (Woodbury, MN: Llewelyn Worldwide, 2016), 7.

4. Michael M. Zanoni, *Healing Resonance Qi Gong and Hamanaleo Meditation: Introductory Comments,* https://docs.wixstatic.com/ugd/9371b9_1f315b1505394b7bb b6ceeb9dc4272a6.pdf (accessed 11/12/2018).

constitution. It is a fundamental substance that is intimately involved with reproduction, growth, and development of the body from birth to death. As we discussed previously, *qi* has been described as the vital, dynamic force that animates the body. It could be considered the current that runs the motor of our metabolism and drives every aspect of our bodily functions. The term *shen* is harder to translate, but it can be thought of as our mind or spirit. Depending upon the context, the word *shen* can mean immortal, god, spirit, mind, or soul.[5]

By practicing qigong we can strengthen the Three Treasures. Because the jing, qi, and shen are inseparable, they each support and fortify the others, leading to better physical and emotional health and well-being.

It is well beyond the scope of this book to have a complete discussion of the metaphysical aspects of qigong.[6] An in-depth understanding of qigong is not necessary for you to begin your practice. What is necessary? You must focus attention on your breath and be aware of the flow of qi as you move your body with intention.

Qigong is a journey. The goal is not perfection but incremental improvement in physical, emotional, and spiritual well-being. Patience and persistence are the keys to receiving the many benefits of qigong.

Benefits of Qigong

Qigong benefits all parts of the body, including all the organ systems and brain.[7] In the following section, we discuss some examples of these benefits.

Nervous System Benefits

Qigong offers huge benefits to our nervous systems, both to the central nervous system and peripheral nervous system. Qigong helps concentra-

---

5. Yang, Jwing-Ming. *The Root of Chinese Qigong: Secrets for Health, Longevity and Enlightenment*, 2nd ed (Wolfeboro, NH: YMAA Publication Center, 1989), 28.

6. For the interested reader, there are many excellent books on this topic listed in the Recommended Reading and Resources section.

7. Dr. Aihan Kuhn, *True Brain Fitness: Preventing Brain Aging through Body Movement* (Wolfeboro, NH: YMAA Publication Center, 2017), 11.

tion, improves mental alertness, and helps to control emotion. It also helps to preserve vision and hearing as the body ages.

Cardiovascular Benefits

Qi is dynamic. It performs like a motor that pushes the blood where it should go. If a person's qi is strong and circulates well in the body, their blood will also circulate well. If a person's qi is stagnant or weak, it will cause blood stagnation which, according to Eastern medical theory, can cause heart disease. Qigong contributes to better heart health by regulating the autonomic nervous system. In particular, these exercises activate the vagus nerve—which is a great way to preserve heart energy, normalize cardiac arrhythmias, and maintain normal blood pressure.

Respiratory Benefits

Through deep and slow breathing, more oxygen goes into the lungs. Deep and slow breathing also activates the parasympathetic (calming) part of the autonomic nervous system. Recall that the nervous system interfaces with the immune system. This process helps the functioning of all cells through proper oxygenation as well as improves defensive energy—which in Western medicine we call the "respiratory immune system"—through modulation of the immune system. The lining of the nose, throat, lungs, gut, and urinary tract all contain immunoglobulin A (IgA). IgA is an antibody in the respiratory tract that protects it from various germs and pathogens and acts as the first line of defense against bacteria and viruses. If the respiratory immune system is strong, immunoglobulin A (IgA) can fight germs, allowing less chance for colds and other respiratory infections to take hold. This is why those who practice qigong generally have fewer illnesses.

Gastrointestinal (GI) Benefits

Qigong can improve stomach and spleen energy, which is related to digestion and absorption. From a Western perspective, qigong regulates the vagus nerve, which also controls digestion. With regular practice, digestive enzymes and digestive movement stay balanced through vagus nerve regulation.

Musculoskeletal Benefits

Once the circulation of the qi and blood are improved, muscles receive more oxygen and blood—the muscles become more resilient, more toned, and stronger. Muscle aging is delayed, and joints become more flexible. Overall, we can maintain a younger body even though we are going through the aging process.

Metabolism and Endocrine System Benefits

Balanced qi also helps regulate the body's organ systems, which helps equilibrate metabolism and the endocrine system. Here again, these benefits are due to the effect that qigong has on our nervous systems. The central and peripheral nervous systems are intimately connected to the endocrine and immune systems. Neuroendocrine-immune dysfunction can explain a variety of Western diagnoses such as chronic fatigue syndrome, also known as myalgic encephalomyelitis.

Immune System Benefits

Qigong maintains normal immune function.[8] We have already spoken about how these exercises can improve respiratory immunity to keep infections at bay. For cancer patients, a healthy immune system can prevent infections during treatment. For those without cancer, a healthy immune system can identify precancerous cells and destroy them.

By balancing the sympathetic and parasympathetic nervous systems, qigong also balances the immune system, so that the immune system is neither too weak nor too strong. A weak immune system will result in recurrent infections. An overly aggressive immune system may result in autoimmune diseases like rheumatoid arthritis. In autoimmune diseases, the immune system turns against the body and attacks normal tissue. Qigong and taiji help keep the immune system balanced.

Other benefits of qigong include delayed aging, improved balance, reduced risk of falling and injury, and improved memory.[9]

---

8. Dr. Aihan Kuhn, *Simple Chinese Medicine: A Beginner's Guide to Natural Healing and Well-Being* (Wolfeboro, NH: YMAA Publication Center, 2009), 137.

9. For further reading, please see Recommended Reading and Resources at the end of this book.

Now it is time to begin your journey and start your qigong practice.

Qigong for the Gut (GI Ailments)

Even if your digestive or metabolic problems resolve with all our previous recommendations, adding qigong into your regular self-care routine will promote a lifetime of well-being.

Do these exercises daily or at least most days of the week and you will see changes. Don't expect a next-day cure, though, because there is no such thing. Qigong is a lifestyle.

Part One: Warm-Up Exercise

1. Shaking the Body

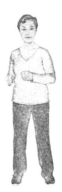

Shake your body at a moderate to fast speed depending on what you feel is right for you.

This movement helps to promote circulation, get your heart rate up, and promote digestive movement.

2. Turn Body Side to Side

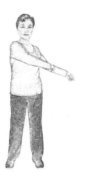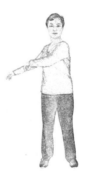

Stand with your feet about shoulder-width apart. Turn your body from side to side in a moderate to fast speed depending on your comfort level. Turn gently. If you turn too vigorously, you may cause misalignment of the joint(s).

This exercise is beneficial to open the nervous system pathway.

3. Shifting Weight, Swing Arms Downward, Backward

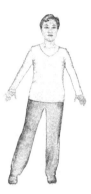

Stand with your feet about shoulder-wide apart and hold your hands at hip height. Shift your weight to the left and press your palms backward in a pulsing motion twenty to thirty times. Move at a moderate to fast speed.

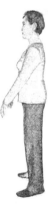

Bring the weight back to the center and relax your palms.

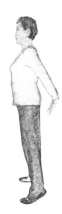

Shift your weight to the right and press your palms downward and backward in a pulsing motion twenty to thirty times.

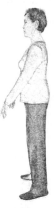

Bring the weight back to the center and relax your palms.

This is a very good exercise to open your energy channel in your arms. It is also good for balance.

4. Turn Body, Moving Arm to Opposite Side

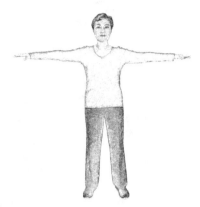

Do this exercise at a moderate to fast speed and keep your feet about shoulder-width apart throughout. Raise your arms to shoulder level.

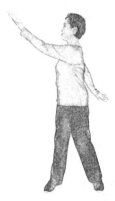

Turn your body to the right and move the left arm to the right and upward while swinging the right arm downward and backward.

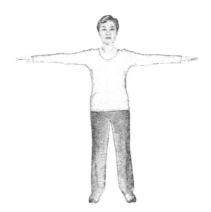

Turn your body back to face forward and move your left arm down and then both arms upward to shoulder level.

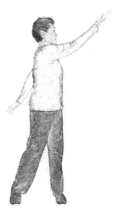

Turn your body to the left and move your right arm to the left and upward while swinging your left arm downward and backward.

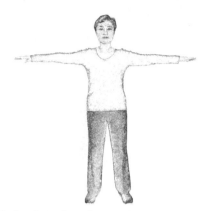

Turn your body back to face forward and move your right arm down and then both arms up to shoulder level.

Repeat this movement twenty to thirty times. In addition to helping to loosen joints, this movement is also helpful in balancing the brain.

5. Waist Rotation

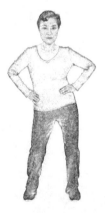
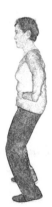

Your feet remain about shoulder-wide apart. Relax your knees and gently circle your waist clockwise eight times, then counterclockwise eight times.

6. Knocking on Leg

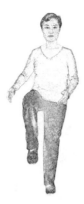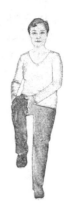

Lift your right leg, and using your palms or fists, knock on your right leg thirty times, from your thigh to your calf, if you can reach that far. If not, only go as far as your lower thigh. Put your leg down.

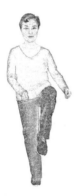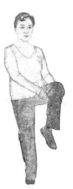

Lift your left leg and, using your palms or fists, knock on your left leg thirty times. Put your leg down.

Part Two: Qigong for the Gut

This short qigong set can help maintain and improve your gut health. Do this set regularly. Once a day is recommended. Do the warm-up exercises described in part one before you begin.

1. Slow Neck Movement

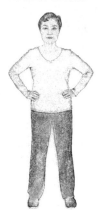 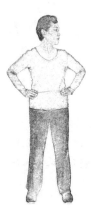

Stand with your feet about shoulder-width apart. Inhale slowly and turn your head to the left.

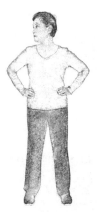 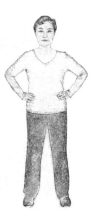

Exhale slowly as you turn your head to face forward.

Inhale slowly and turn your head to the right. Exhale slowly as you turn head back to center.

Repeat one to three more times to each side.

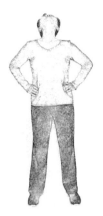 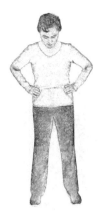

Inhale and move your chin upward. Stretch the front neck muscles. Exhale and move your head downward.

Repeat this movement three more times.

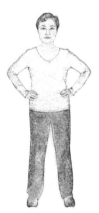 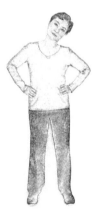

Inhale and return your head to the upright position. Exhale and tilt your head toward your left shoulder.

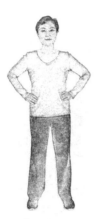 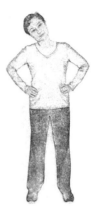

Inhale and return your head to the upright position. Exhale and tilt your head to the right.

Repeat these movements two to three times.

2. Pushing Horseman

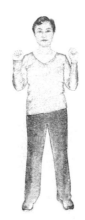

Stand with your feet about shoulder-width apart. Bend your arms, and place your hands next to your shoulders. Make light fists. Inhale.

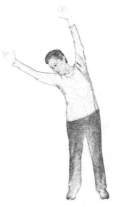

Exhale and lean your upper body to the right, and at the same time push your hands upward and open your fists. Look to the right and downward.

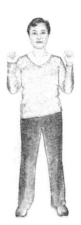

Inhale and return to the position with your fists next to your shoulders.

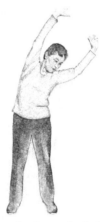

Exhale and lean your upper body to the left and at the same time push your hands upward and open your fists. Look to the left and downward.

Repeat the whole sequence four to eight times.

3. Rotational Arm Stretching

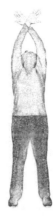

Stand with your feet about shoulder-width apart. Overlap your hands in front of you. With arms straight, but not locked, inhale and slowly raise your hands over your head. Your eyes follow your hands as they move upward.

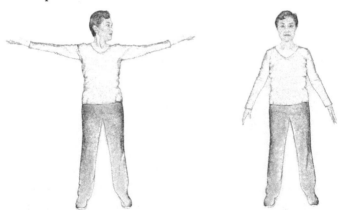

Exhale, separate your hands and move them down to the sides of your body, keeping the arms straight but not locked. Your eyes follow your left hand to the side. Lower your hands to hip height and face forward.

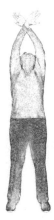

Again overlap hands in front of you. Inhale slowly and raise your hands above your head with the arms straight.

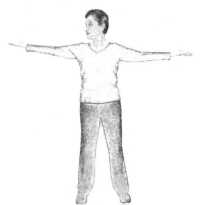 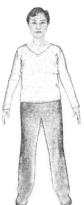

Exhale, separate your hands, and move them down to the sides of your body, keeping the arms straight but not locked. Your eyes follow your right hand to the side. Lower your hands to hip height and face forward.

Repeat the whole sequence four to eight times.

Important Note: When your arms are above your head, try to straighten them unless you have a problem. When you separate your arms and move them downward, try to open your arms as wide as you can. Your breaths need to be deep, slow, and smooth.

4. Angel Wings

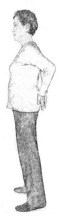

Stand with your feet about shoulder-wide apart. Place both hands near your lower back, palms facing the sacroiliac joint but not touching the body.

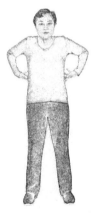
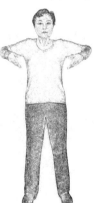

Inhale and slowly raise your shoulders as high as you can, as you move your hands upward and then up the sides of the body.

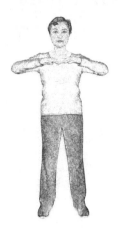 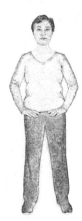

Exhale, and slowly move your hands to the front of your body. Then relax your shoulders and slowly move your palms downward.

Repeat this movement four to eight times.

5. Holding Sky, Swing Body to Side

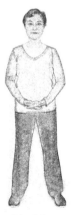

Stand with your feet about shoulder-width apart. Interlock your fingers in front of your body.

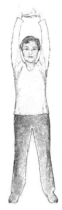

Inhale while raising your hands up above your head until your arms are straight and your palms face upward.

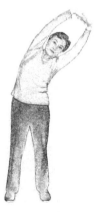

Exhale and slowly bend your upper body to the left.

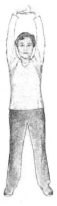

Inhale and return to the upright position.

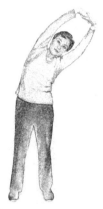

Bend your body to the left again.

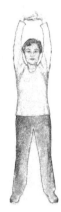

Inhale and return to the upright position.

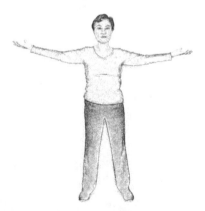

Exhale, separate your hands, and lower them to hip level.

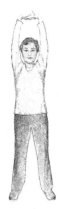

Inhale and raise your hands up above the head until your arms are straight and your palms face upward.

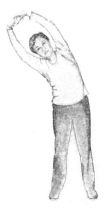

Exhale and slowly bend your upper body to the right.

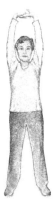

Inhale and return to the upright position.

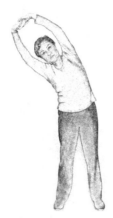

Bend your body to the right again.

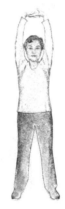

Inhale and return to the upright position.

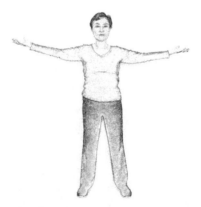

Exhale, separate your hands, and lower them to hip level.

6. Swing Arms and Upper Body

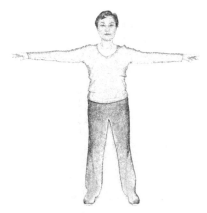

Stand with your feet about shoulder-width apart. Inhale and move your arms to shoulder level.

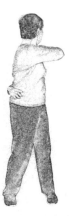

Exhale, turn your upper body to the left, and swing your arms to the left, placing your right hand over your left shoulder and your left hand behind your back, palms facing outward. Turn your head over your right shoulder and look behind you.

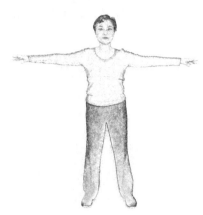

Inhale and move your arms to shoulder level.

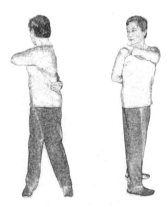

Exhale, turn your upper body to the right and swing your arms to the right, left hand over your right shoulder and your right hand behind your lower back, palms facing outward. Turn your head over your right shoulder and look to the back.

Repeat this movement for a total of eight times.

Important note: Do not move your feet when you turn your body and swing your arms. Turn your body and your head in the same direction. Turn as far as you can without hurting yourself. Your eyes should follow in the same direction as you turn your body. Relax your waist and your whole body.

7. Cover Knees, Stretching Leg

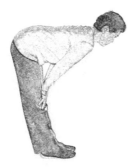

Stand with your feet together. Place both hands on your knees and gently push your hips backward. The goal is to lengthen your back.

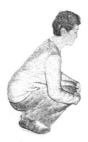

Slowly bend both knees and go down into a squatting position with the feet flat. It will feel like you are squeezing your abdomen. Hold this position for one breath. If you cannot squat with the feet flat you may lift your heels.

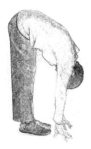

Place your hands on the top of your feet or on the floor, and slowly raise your hips as you straighten your legs.

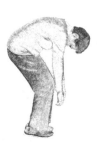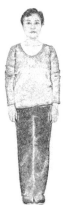

Slowly roll the upper body to an upright position. Then relax the body.

Repeat four times.

Important Note: Try to keep your hands on your feet or the floor as you raise your hips and straighten your legs. If you cannot keep your hands on your feet or the floor you can modify the position of your hands according to your abilities.

8. Reaching Feet

Stand with your feet together. Interlock your fingers in front of your body. Inhale and raise your interlocked hands above your head. Keep your eyes on your hands. Rotate your palms so they face upward when the arms are straight.

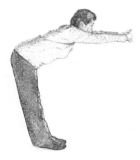

Exhale and slowly bend forward. Keep your arms and your cervical and thoracic vertebrae straight.

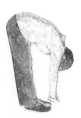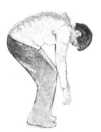

Continue to move downward until your hands reach your feet. When your hands are as low as they can go, unlock your fingers and allow your hands to relax. Let your arms hang with your fingers pointing toward the floor. Relax your shoulders, arms, neck, and head. Let gravity gently release the tension in your neck. Take two slow breaths.

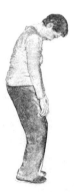

Roll your body back up to an upright position.

Repeat a total of four times.

9. Look at the Moon

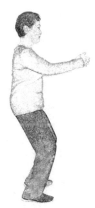

Stand with your feet about shoulder-width apart. With yours knees slightly bent, place your arms in front of your chest like you are holding a big ball and inhale.

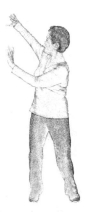 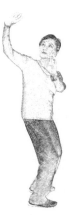

Exhale as you turn your body to the right. As you turn, move your arms to the upper right and turn your palms to face the upper right position. Look to the upper right.

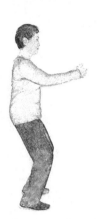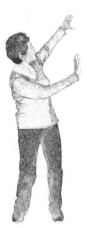

Inhale and turn to face forward. Your arms return to the position of holding a big ball.

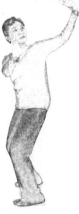

Exhale as you turn your body to the left. As you turn, move your arms to the upper left, and turn your palms to face the upper left. Look to the upper left.

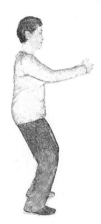

Inhale, and turn to face forward. Your arms return to the position of holding a big ball.

Repeat a total of four times.

10. Abdominal Massage

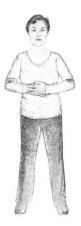

Stand with your feet about shoulder-width apart. Overlap your hands and place them over the upper abdomen.

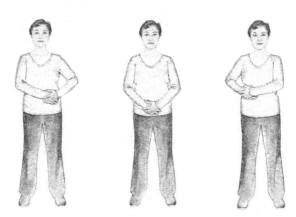

With a gentle pressure, move your hands in a full circle around your abdomen, eight times in one direction, then change to the opposite direction and circle eight times. Move from the left abdomen to the lower abdomen, to the right abdomen, to the upper abdomen, and then circle in the opposite direction.

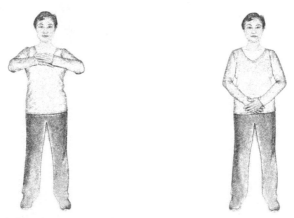

Finish by placing your hands over the upper chest and inhale. Exhale and push downward along the middle line of the body back to the abdomen.

11. Ending

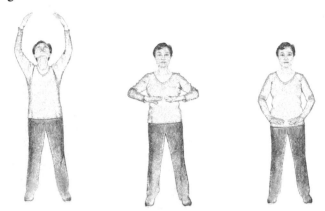

Stand with your feet about shoulder-wide apart. Take a deep breath and raise your arms from your sides to above your head. Exhale and move your hands down in the front of your body.

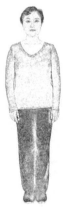

Bring your feet together and relax the entire body.

You may repeat the entire set if you have time. It is short enough that you can do it during a break at work. If you can do it every day, that will be ideal for your healing. You may get unexpected benefits, which would be a bonus for your hard work.

Good luck with your daily practice. For video information, please visit www.draihankuhn.com.

CHAPTER 7

General Principles of Self-Healing

ULTIMATELY, the successful management of all diseases including gastrointestinal disease, diabetes, and obesity, depends upon consistent self-care. Even if you are taking medications for these conditions, you must be attentive to your body, mind, and spirit on a daily basis. Medications must be taken regularly without skipping doses, and doctors' appointments should be kept. There is a lot that your health-care provider can do, from arriving at a correct diagnosis to arranging specialty and support services.

But there is even more that you can do for yourself. We all know that eating nutritious foods, not smoking, exercising regularly, sleeping adequately, and managing stress levels can lead to a healthier life. In fact, the World Health Organization (WHO) and Centers for Disease Control (CDC) have determined that by exercising more, eating better, and not smoking, 40 percent of cancers and 80 percent of adult-onset diabetes and heart disease could be prevented.[1] Sleep deprivation and life stress have each been shown to contribute to the incidence of chronic illness, so sleeping well and managing your stress can decrease your risk of such diseases.

Taking care of yourself requires determination. Every day you will be faced with choices about what foods to buy, how to cook them, how much to eat, and how to exercise and for how long. You also make choices about whether to go to sleep at a reasonable hour or stay up and surf the internet. You choose whether to manage your stress by meditative practices or

---

1. Kenneth Thorpe and Jonathan Lever, "Prevention: The Answer to Curbing Chronically High Health Care Costs," May 24, 2011, http://www.kaiserhealthnews.org/Columns/2011/May/052411thorpelever.aspx.

dangerous habits such as smoking or excessive alcohol consumption. Every decision you make matters. Your doctor can give you advice but, ultimately, you must decide for yourself and act on those decisions. No one else can do it for you.

If you have already established these healthy habits, congratulations! You are stacking the odds in your favor. The likelihood that you will develop a lifestyle-related chronic illness is at least half what it would be otherwise. As we have seen, even conditions like heart disease can be improved through lifestyle modification.

If you feel there is room for improvement in the way you eat, exercise, and manage your stress, now is the time to gear up and get going. In our first book, *True Wellness: How to Combine the Best of Western and Eastern Medicine for Optimal Health*, we devoted a whole chapter to the process of change, setting goals, and taking action to achieve those objectives. As mentioned earlier, we have found that one of the most useful tools you can use to establish new habits is a checklist. There is nothing particularly glamorous or high-tech about a checklist, but for many people, it is invaluable. With a checklist, you can see concretely what you have or have not done during the course of your week. If you plan to practice qigong three times a week, you can see as the days pass whether you will meet that goal. If you are honest, you will see the number of times you meditated or went to the gym, how many vegetables you ate, or how much water you drank. Many people, when they start using a checklist, are astonished at their own lapses. We often convince ourselves that we are doing all we can to achieve optimal health, when really we are falling short of the mark. This sort of wishful thinking is very common.

The beauty of a checklist is that it gives you a systematic way of changing your behavior and developing consistency. The checklist has become integral in air-traffic safety and in hospital operating rooms. Its use has improved outcomes in these industries where lives hang in the balance. It is not being too melodramatic to say that both the quality and quantity of your years on Earth depend on establishing habits that maximize your physical, emotional, and spiritual health.

Decades of medical research show that most chronic illnesses are lifestyle driven and that the underlying physiological problem in these conditions is chronic inflammation. Many studies demonstrate that eating a minimally processed plant-based diet; meditating; practicing qigong, taiji, or yoga; exercising regularly; and getting adequate sleep all decrease chronic inflammation. Using the True Wellness Checklist can effectively support your shift toward healthy lifestyle, decrease chronic inflammation, and reduce your risk of developing many chronic conditions.

The True Wellness Checklist

Instructions for Use
The True Wellness Checklist is a compilation of recommended actions that are associated with optimal health. These actions form the basis of disease prevention in both Eastern and Western medical systems. Meditation, qigong, cardiovascular exercise, and resistance training should be incorporated into everyone's healing plan. Optimizing your sleep can improve your physical and emotional health. Sleep has an enormous effect on all chronic conditions. This is why we have included in this custom version of the True Wellness Checklist measures you can take to improve the quality and quantity of your sleep.

Many people have food sensitivities, allergies, or individual preferences; therefore, the dietary recommendations on the checklist form the essentials of a vegan regimen. You can add servings of meat, fish, or dairy depending on your tastes or requirements. The majority of your food should be plant based. If you do eat animal products, your plate should be filled three-quarters with plants and only one-quarter with animal protein. Choose whole foods over processed foods. Minimize sweets, but on occasion enjoy chocolate made of at least 70 percent cacao.

Approximate Serving Sizes	
Vegetables	1 cup raw vegetables, ½ cup cooked vegetables
Fruit	1 medium piece of raw fruit, ½ cup canned fruit, ¼ cup dried fruit
Nuts	1/3 cup
Beans/Legumes	½ cup cooked
Whole Grains	1 slice of bread, ½ cup cooked grains, 1 ounce dry cereal
Red Meat, Poultry	cooked, roughly the same size as a deck of cards

Fish	uncooked, 8 ounces (no more than 3x/week due to heavy metals)
Dairy	1 cup of yogurt, 1 cup of milk, 2 ounces of cheese
Eggs	1 egg
Oils	extra virgin olive oil (cooking/dressings), flax-seed oil (dressings)

True Wellness Checklist

Daily Practice	Day 1	Day 2	Day 3	Day 4	Day 5	Day 6	Day 7
sleep							
• Wake up at the same time every day	☐	☐	☐	☐	☐	☐	☐
• Meditate daily	☐	☐	☐	☐	☐	☐	☐
• No caffeine after 3:00 p.m.	☐	☐	☐	☐	☐	☐	☐
• No naps after 3:00 p.m.	☐	☐	☐	☐	☐	☐	☐
• Exercise no later than 3 hours before bed	☐	☐	☐	☐	☐	☐	
• No electronics 1–2 hours before bed	☐	☐	☐	☐	☐	☐	☐
• Keep bedroom cool and dark	☐	☐	☐	☐	☐	☐	☐
• Go to bed at the same time every night, if sleepy	☐	☐	☐	☐	☐	☐	☐
• If not asleep in 15 minutes, get up and meditate, then lie down again when sleepy*	☐	☐	☐	☐	☐	☐	☐
food							
• Eat during a 24-hour window	☐	☐	☐	☐	☐	☐	☐
• Vegetables (4–6 servings daily)	☐	☐	☐	☐	☐	☐	☐
• Fruit (3–4 servings daily)	☐	☐	☐	☐	☐	☐	☐
• Nuts (1/3 cup daily)	☐	☐	☐	☐	☐	☐	☐
• Beans/Legumes (1–2 servings daily)	☐	☐	☐	☐	☐	☐	☐
• Grains (3–4 servings daily)	☐	☐	☐	☐	☐	☐	☐
• Water (8 glasses daily)	☐	☐	☐	☐	☐	☐	☐
• Protein of choice (1–3 servings)							
move-ment							
• Cardiovascular exercise (2–5x/week)	☐	☐	☐	☐	☐	☐	☐
• Resistance training (2–5x/week)	☐	☐	☐	☐	☐	☐	☐
• Qigong or Tai Chi (5–7x/week)	☐	☐	☐	☐	☐	☐	☐
fun							
• *At least* one 15-minute activity every day, simply for your own enjoyment	☐	☐	☐	☐	☐	☐	☐

Conclusion

"Knowing is not enough, we must apply. Willing is not enough, we must do."

—Bruce Lee

TAKING RESPONSIBILITY for your health can feel like a daunting task. Change can be scary, even if it leads to a positive outcome. We have presented you with loads of information to help you achieve your goals, but the rest is up to you. Some people are able to tackle problems head-on, make sweeping lifestyle changes, and make them stick. In our experience, most people need more support. You may be one of those people and that is perfectly fine. Acknowledging the necessity for assistance is the first step in making change. Speak to your family and friends about your plans and see how you can involve them in your healing strategy. Arrange to meet for walks, get your spouse and children into the kitchen, or sign up for a qigong class together. Social interactions augment the beneficial effects of these healthy activities.

Sudden large changes are often unsustainable. This is why many individuals fail to alter habits that are damaging to their health. The best way to avoid this pitfall is to make these changes little by little. Research into how people make change has shown that small, easy, incremental adjustments are more likely to lead to lasting success. Think of yourself as an infant learning to walk with baby steps, one foot at a time.

For people with significant health problems, getting this process started can be problematic. Maybe you can't get around the block. Maybe you have suffered from digestive problems for years and seen doctor after doctor without result. Maybe you have tried every weight loss plan out there only to regain every pound you lost. As obvious as this sounds, you have to start from where you are. To use a running analogy, the goal may be to complete a marathon, but you must honestly assess your current exercise tolerance and gradually increase your time, distance, and intensity. This same thinking applies to every aspect of health.

The True Wellness Checklist is a reminder of the goals we strive to reach. If you are in the position, as so many are, where you need to make significant modifications to all the categories listed you may feel disheartened if you try to fix everything at once. Set yourself up for success by making one change at a time. You can choose the category, but keep the change small and simple. For example, with respect to food, eat one more serving of vegetables than you normally would each day. Each day you do so, check that box and give yourself credit! After several days of completing this new change, reward yourself in a healthy way, and make another small change. If you put on your running shoes and walk out onto your porch and back, check the exercise box. If you turn off your electronics even thirty minutes before going to bed, check the sleep box. If you do one qigong exercise or take three deep breaths, check those boxes, too. If you are focusing on the Four Phase Elimination Diet, avoid only one problematic food group to start, but be consistent. Even with these tiny changes, you will start to feel more energized and encouraged. Pay attention to the process and you will eventually reach the goal. Science has shown that repeated action coupled with an appropriate reward will increase your motivation and create an automatic response. This is how you create a habit. So, feel free to tailor the True Wellness Checklist to meet your needs. Be patient, but be persistent. You want these changes to last a lifetime.

Sleep, food, and movement are the building blocks of optimal health, but don't forget about fun. Make sure that you have activities in your life that you enjoy and find relaxing. If you find you are unable to relax, your underlying chronic stress may be the cause. If you are living or working in an environment that constantly activates your fight-or-flight response, you may have great difficulty healing.

Who you are sharing dinner with is more important that *what* you are eating. Your physical and emotional safety is more important than whether you can run a marathon. While everyone needs to earn a living, consider whether your job is significantly contributing to your chronic stress and health problems. Think about changes you can make to protect yourself and prevent your condition from worsening.

These are all very serious issues and we recommend that you seek help from your healthcare provider if you are in this position. We both feel strongly that the patient and the health-care provider must work as a team. If you don't feel comfortable sharing these concerns with your doctor, find another primary care provider or therapist with whom you can discuss your concerns. Your input matters. Engagement in your own healing creates equilibrium within this partnership and advances your healing.

As you move forward you will see that more than your individual health hangs in the balance. You will be a role model for those around you. Your friends, your parents, your coworkers, and your children will all notice the positive changes you will achieve in your physical, mental, and emotional health. You may inspire others to tackle their own health concerns. More importantly, you may encourage others, particularly the children in your life, to adopt habits that will prevent them from falling ill in the first place.

No matter where you start your journey, the positive actions you take now will change your life. The practices and behaviors we have described affect the neurology, gene expression, and biochemistry of the body and microbiome, effectively restoring health and preventing disease. In your quest for true wellness, keep an open mind and take advantage of all that Western and Eastern medicine can offer. Consistently weaving Eastern therapies into Western care will give you an advantage when setbacks occur, as they inevitably will. You will have the tools in place to more easily weather the storm and gain confidence in your capabilities and increasing resilience. This is the beauty of integrative medicine. Whether you are seeking optimal digestive health, glucose control, or weight loss, each component we have discussed supports the other, magnifying the positive effects synergistically. If these principles are consistently applied, your actions *will* make a difference.

We wish you every success on your journey.

Acknowledgements

We are continually appreciative of the enthusiasm and encouragement we receive from the great team at YMAA Publication Center. Publisher, David Ripianzi, and editor, Leslie Takao, always offer guidance with humor and grace. Getting a book from a concept to something tangible, either hardcopy or digital, requires hard work and attention to detail. We are supported in this manner by not only David and Leslie, but by production manager Tim Comrie, illustrator and designer Axie Breen, copyeditor Doran Hunter, and publicist Barbara Langley. Thank you, all!

Michael M. Zanoni, PhD, has been generously sharing his time and knowledge of Eastern medicine, qigong, and meditation with thousands of his patients and students. His background in biochemistry and biomedicine give him keen insights into the ways in which Eastern and Western medicine can be safely and effectively combined. We are grateful to Dr. Zanoni for bringing his vast experience in East/West integration to the writing of the foreword for this book.

Individually, we would like to acknowledge the following people:

AK: I want to take this opportunity to thank my dear supporters of my teaching, book writing, and my non-profit work. I appreciate the support and kindness of Marshall Garland, Gail Pettit, Patricia Gerlek, Kate Orav, Jennifer Cable, and Pam Vlakakis. In addition, I want to thank all my fans and readers who give me valuable feedback that helps me to improve my work.

CK: I am indebted to Dr. Rosa Schnyer for her suggestions and advice. Her guidance has allowed me to broaden my understanding of the history and foundations of acupuncture, and I am most appreciative of the time and attention that she has spent reading our work. I would also like to thank my family, yet again, for their love, patience, and support.

And last, but far from least, we would like to thank our patients with whom we share this endlessly fascinating journey.

Glycemic Index and Glycemic Load

The glycemic index is a measure of how quickly a food is digested into simple sugars within a specific time. The index uses a standardized amount of white bread as its reference point because it is metabolized very quickly and causes sudden increases in blood sugar levels. One slice of white bread is assigned a value of 100. The glycemic index compares how an equivalent amount of other foods affects blood sugar levels in the same amount of time. The glycemic index of a food is assigned a number between 1 and 100 based on how quickly it raises blood sugar values compared to white bread. For example, an apple has a low glycemic index value because it causes a lower rise in blood sugar levels compared to white bread in the same amount of time. In general, low, medium, and high glycemic index (GI) values are grouped as below:

Low GI < 55
Medium GI = 56-69
High GI > 70

Glycemic load uses the glycemic index but goes a step further. It also takes into account the amount of carbohydrates that a food contains in a typical serving. When you compare foods, you find that those foods with a low glycemic index will also have a low glycemic load, but those with a high glycemic index may have either a high glycemic load or a low glycemic load once the available carbohydrate content is considered. The available carbohydrate content means the usable carbohydrates that are left once the fiber has been removed. Using an equation to determine the glycemic load factors in the carbohydrate content, so it gives you a more accurate prediction of how a particular food will affect your blood sugar levels. Fortunately, there are many lists available that can give you the glycemic index and load of a specific food, so you don't have to do all that math!

Foods that have rapidly digestible sugar but also a high water content will have a high glycemic index value but a low glycemic load. This is because there is relatively little sugar in an average serving of the food. Fat also plays a role in how quickly a food is digested, but this is not incorporated in the basic glycemic load equation. Let's run the conversion from glycemic index to glycemic load using watermelon as an example.

The general conversion equation is:

$$\text{Glycemic load of a food} = \frac{(\text{Glycemic index of that food x grams of available carbohydrates it contains})}{100}$$

There are different levels of glycemic load, classified as low, medium, and high. These classifications reflect how quickly and how high a particular food will elevate your blood sugar. The ranges of these levels of glycemic load (GL) are as follows:

Low GL < 10

Moderate GL < 11–19

High GL > 20

So, for 120 grams (roughly 4 ounces) of watermelon:
- The glycemic index of 120 grams of watermelon is 72.
- The amount of available carbohydrates in this much watermelon is 6 grams.

Therefore, the glycemic load of 120 grams of watermelon is:

$$\text{Glycemic Load} = \frac{(72 \times 6)}{100} = 100$$

This means that watermelon will not raise your blood sugar levels too high or too quickly. Low glycemic load foods tend to keep blood sugar levels on an even keel, without any huge spikes. This is beneficial because your body does not have to produce a lot of insulin to deal with the excess sugar. Then it is less likely that your cells would become resistant to insulin and your risk of developing type 2 diabetes is lower.

An example of glycemic index/glycemic load tables can be found at the Harvard Health website:

https://www.health.harvard.edu/diseases-and-conditions/glycemic-index-and-glycemic-load-for-100-foods,

As with all dietary changes, common sense should prevail. This information is presented for you to think about what you are eating and how it affects your body. It is not meant to endorse low glycemic load diets as the only way to eat.

Recommended Reading and Resources

Websites

American Academy of Medical Acupuncture, https://www.medicalacupuncture.org/ Find-an-Acupuncturist

National Certification Commission for Acupuncture and Oriental Medicine, https://www.nccaom.org/find-a-practitioner-directory

National Institutes of Health, U.S. National Library of Medicine—Medline Plus, https://medlineplus.gov/digestivesystem.html

Satchin Panda, PhD., Salk Institute, https://www.mycircadianclock.org

Tai Chi & Qi Gong Healing Institute www.taichihealing.org

Dr. Subhas Ganguli, Gastroenterologist www.foodasprevention.com

Books

Aujla, Rupy. *Eat to Beat Illness: 80 Simple, Delicious Recipes Inspired by the Science of Food as Medicine.* New York: HarperOne, 2019.

Blaser, Martin J. *Missing Microbes: How the Overuse of Antibiotics Is Fueling Our Modern Plagues.* New York: Henry Holt and Company, 2014.

Buettner, Dan. *The Blue Zones: Lessons for Living Longer from the People Who've Lived the Longest,* National Geographic: Washington DC, 2008.

Chatterjee, Rangan. *Feel Better in 5: Your Daily Plan to Feel Great for Life.* London: Penguin Life, 2019.

Chatterjee, Rangan. *How to Make Disease Disappear.* New York: HarperCollins, 2018.

Chatterjee, Rangan. *The Stress Solution: The 4 Steps to Reset Your Body, Mind, Relationships, and Purpose.* London: Penguin Life, 2018.

Clear, James. *Atomic Habits: An Easy and Proven Way to Break Bad Habits and Build Good Ones.* New York: Avery Penguin, 2018.

Cohen, Kenneth. *The Way of Qigong: The Art and Science of Chinese Energy Healing.* New York: Ballantine Books, 1997.

Doidge, Norman. *The Brain That Changes Itself.* New York: Viking/Penguin, 2007.

Doidge, Norman. *The Brain's Way of Healing.* New York: Penguin, 2015.

Greger, Michael. *How Not to Diet: The Groundbreaking Science of Healthy, Permanent Weight Loss.* New York: Flatiron, 2019.

Harris, Dan. *10% Happier: How I Tamed the Voice in My Head, Reduced Stress without Losing My Edge, and Found Self-Help That Actually Works—A True Story.* New York: HarperCollins, 2014.

Helms, Joseph. *Getting to Know You: A Physician Explains How Acupuncture Helps You Be the Best You.* Berkeley, CA: M.A.P. Medical Acupuncture Publishers, 2007.

Hyman, Mark. *Food: What the Heck Should I Eat?* New York: Little, Brown Spark, 2018.

Jonas, Wayne. *How Healing Works: Get Well and Stay Well Using Your Hidden Power to Heal.* New York: Penguin Random House, 2018.

Kaptchuk, Ted. *The Web That Has No Weaver: Understanding Chinese Medicine.* New York: McGraw-Hill, 2000.

Keown, Daniel. *The Spark in the Machine: How the Science of Acupuncture Explains the Mysteries of Western Medicine.* London: Singing Dragon, 2014.

Kuhn, Aihan. *Natural Healing with Qigong: Therapeutic Qigong.* Wolfeboro: YMAA Publication Center, 2004.

Kuhn, Aihan. *Simple Chinese Medicine: A Beginner's Guide to Natural Healing and Well-Being.* Wolfeboro, NH: YMAA Publication Center, 2009.

Kuhn, Aihan. *Tai Chi in 10 Weeks: Beginner's Guide: A Proven Step-by-Step Plan for Integrating the Physical and Psychological Benefits of Tai Chi into Your Life.* Wolfeboro, NH: YMAA Publication Center, 2017.

Kurosu, Catherine, and Aihan Kuhn. *True Wellness: How to Combine the Best of Western and Eastern Medicine for Optimal Health.* Wolfeboro, NH: YMAA Publication Center, 2018.

Lee, Jennie. *Breathing Love: Meditation in Action.* Woodbury, MN: Llewellyn Worldwide, 2018.

Lee, Jennie. *True Yoga: Practicing with the Yoga Sutras for Happiness and Spiritual Fulfillment.* Woodbury, MN: Llewellyn Worldwide, 2016.

Mayer, Emeran. *The Mind-Gut Connection: How the Hidden Conversation within Our Bodies Impacts Our Mood, Our Choices, and Our Overall Health.* New York: HarperWave, 2016.

Mullin, Gerard E. and Kathie Madonna Swift, *The Inside Tract: Your Good Gut Guide to Great Digestive Health.* New York: Rodale, 2011.

Mullin, Gerard E., *The Gut Balance Revolution.* New York: Rodale, 2015.

Perlmutter, David. *Brain Maker: The Power of Gut Microbes to Heal and Protect Your Brain—for Life.* New York: Little, Brown Spark, 2015.

Ruscio, Michael. *Healthy Gut, Healthy You: The Personalized Plan to Transform Your Health from the Inside Out.* Las Vegas: The Ruscio Institute, 2018.

Scheid, Volker, and Hugh MacPherson, editors. *Integrating East Asian Medicine into Contemporary Health Care.* Edinburgh: Churchill Livingstone, Elsevier, 2012.

Walker, Matthew. *Why We Sleep: Unlocking the Power of Sleep and Dreams.* New York: Scribner, 2017.

Weil, Andrew. *You Can't Afford to Get Sick: Your Guide to Optimum Health and Health Care.* New York: Plume, 2009.

Yang, Jwing-Ming. *The Root of Chinese Qigong: Secrets for Health, Longevity, and Enlightenment.* 2nd ed. Wolfeboro, NH: YMAA Publication Center, 1989.

Glossary

acupuncture. A system of medicine that involves inserting fine metal needles into specific anatomic locations to treat a variety of illnesses and conditions. Derived from the Latin *acus* (needle) and puncture.

allostasis. The physiologic process of maintaining stability during stressful life events that tax a person's metabolism, intellect, or psyche.

American Academy of Medical Acupuncture (AAMA). A society, founded in 1987, of medical doctors (MDs) and osteopaths (DOs) who have undergone training in acupuncture in order to incorporate this modality into conventional health care.

American Board of Medical Acupuncture (ABMA). An independent entity within the AAMA, established in 2000, to conduct examinations of candidates seeking certification in Medical Acupuncture in order to maintain high standards for the profession.

American Medical Association (AMA). A professional association of medical doctors (MDs) and osteopaths (DOs) founded in 1847. The stated mission of the AMA is to "promote the art and science of medicine and the betterment of public health."

autonomic nervous system. The branch of the nervous system of the body that operates without conscious thought and governs the internal organs, bloods vessels, pupils, and sweat, salivary, and digestive glands. The divisions of the autonomic nervous system are the sympathetic, parasympathetic, and enteric nervous systems.

Ben Cao Gang Mu (Compendium of Materia Medica). An encyclopedic medical volume detailing the herbs and other substances used in Chinese medicine. Written in the sixteenth century CE by Li Shi-Zhen, a prominent physician in the Ming dynasty.

Buddhism. A philosophical practice that developed out of the teachings of Siddhartha Gautama in the fifth century BCE and from northeastern India through Asia and globally. Gautama became known as Buddha and taught that life is full of suffering, but suffering could be overcome by developing wisdom, integrity, and awareness.

celiac disease. A chronic disorder in which the ingestion of gluten causes an immune reaction that damages the lining of the small intestine causing many physical symptoms and poor absorption of nutrients.

Circadian rhythm. The body's natural biological and sleep-wake cycle that repeats approximately every twenty-four hours.

Confucianism. The teachings of Confucius, which emphasize correct behavior of the institutions and individuals within society as well as the cultivation of knowledge and good judgment.

Confucius. Chinese philosopher, political figure, and educator who lived during the fifth and sixth centuries, BCE, whose teachings are known as Confucianism.

Crohn's disease. A type of inflammatory bowel disease (IBD) that can cause chronic inflammation in the digestive tract, most commonly in the ileum of the small intestine, and can manifest outside of the gastrointestinal tract.

dan tian. Reservoirs of qi located in the upper, middle, and lower parts of the body and connect with the extraordinary channels.

Dao De Ching. A Chinese text regarding the philosophy of Daoism, attributed to Laozi (see Daoism), which may actually be a compilation of works by later authors.

Daoism. Also known as Taoism. The doctrine of living in harmony with the natural order of the universe, ascribed to the teachings of Laozi, a Chinese philosopher who lived during the sixth century BCE.

diabetes mellitus. A disease in which a person's ability to process glucose is impaired, either by a lack of insulin (type-1 diabetes mellitus) or due to problems transporting glucose from the blood stream into the cells (type 2 diabetes mellitus).

digestion. The process by which nutrients are extracted from ingested food.

Eastern medicine. A system of medicine that arose in Asia that makes use of herbal remedies, acupuncture, meditation, qigong, and taiji to improve health. Also known as East Asian medicine or Oriental medicine.

Elimination Diet. The method of identifying foods that may be causing health problems by eliminating the suspected foods, then reintroducing them into the diet very slowly, usually one food every added back every seventy-two hours.

enteric nervous system. A division of the autonomic nervous system found throughout the gastrointestinal tract that can act independently, relaying sensory input to the brain, modulating the process of digestion, and interacting with the gut microbiome. Also known as the "second brain."

epigenetics. The study of inherited or newly displayed characteristics that are a result of the way in which genes are expressed rather than an actual change in organism's genetic code.

extraordinary channels. Acupuncture channels that act as conduits between the dan tian and the twelve principal channels.

Five Phases. The cosmological scheme that describes interactions among natural phenomena, such as the changing of the seasons, developed in ancient China millennia ago and used in astrology, military strategy, and medicine. Also referred to as the Five Elements. (See Wu Xing.)

FODMAPs. Foods that contain particular types of carbohydrates and sugars that are not well absorbed when the gut lining is inflamed, causing abdominal pain and distention. As a group, these foods are known as FODMAPs, an acronym for Fermentable Oligo-, Di-, and Monosaccharides and Polyols.

functional magnetic resonance imaging (fMRI). An imaging technique that employs magnetic and radio waves, used to determine which areas of the brain are most active at the time of the study.

gastroesophageal reflux disease (GERD). A digestive disorder in which stomach acid comes up into the lower part of the esophagus, which is an abnormal occurrence.

gastrointestinal tract. The organs involved in the act of digestion of food including the mouth, espophagus, stomach, small and large intestines, and rectum.

gene. A protein sequence that codes for a molecule that has a specific function within a living organism.

ghrelin. A hormone that is secreted mostly by the stomach and stimulates appetite.

glycemic index. A measure of the rate at which particular foods increase blood sugar levels.

Hua Tuo. Famed second-century CE Chinese physician and surgeon who also developed longevity exercises called Five Animal Qigong.

Huang Di Nei Jing (The Yellow Emperor's Classic of Internal Medicine). An ancient Chinese medical text written approximately during the Han dynasty (206 BCE–220 CE).

inflammatory bowel disease (IBD). A term used to describe diseases caused by chronic inflammation of the gastrointestinal tract.

integrative medicine. A branch of conventional Western medicine that is patient-centered and incorporates techniques from other medical systems for which there is good evidence of safety and efficacy.

irritable bowel syndrome (IBS). A functional disorder of the bowels thought to result from gut-brain miscommunication.

Journal of the American Medical Association (JAMA). A peer-reviewed medical journal published by the AMA containing research papers, reviews, and editorials that relate to the field of medicine.

Laozi. A Chinese philosopher who lived during the sixth century BCE and developed the doctrine of living in harmony with the natural order of the universe. This doctrine is known as Daoism or Taoism.

leptin. A hormone that is secreted by fat cells and acts in the hypothalamus of the brain to suppress appetite.

licensed acupuncturist (LAc). Designation given to a person who has received a license to practice acupuncture from a state medical or professional licensing board. To qualify, that person must have completed a specific amount of training and passed certifying examinations in acupuncture and Eastern medicine.

metabolism. The biochemical processes involved in the conversion of food to energy in order to support the functions of life.

microbiome. The microorganisms found in various parts of the body or particular environment.

mind-body medicine. A group of therapeutic practices that engage the mind's capacity to influence bodily functions; examples of these techniques include meditation, relaxation, biofeedback, and hypnosis.

National Certification Commission for Acupuncture and Oriental Medicine (NCCAOM). A non-profit organization established in 1982 to certify competency of acupuncturists, herbologists, and bodyworkers of Eastern medical disciplines in the United States. The NCCAOM is also involved with recertification, examination development, and continuing education.

neuroplasticity. The ability of the brain to form new connections and pathways in response to learning or training; also known as brain plasticity.

parasympathetic nervous system. The division of the autonomic nervous system that controls the relaxation response and digestion, commonly referred to as the "rest and digest" response.

peristalsis. The involuntary movements of the gastrointestinal tract muscles that move food through the different areas in the tract and aid in the process of digestion.

placebo effect. A positive, unexpected benefit seen following administration of a placebo. Attributed to the recipient's expectation of benefit, considered a mind-body interaction that activates the recipient's innate ability to heal.

placebo. A substance or intervention that has no active ingredient or expected benefit.

post-heaven qi. Eastern medicine term for energy (qi) extracted by the body from food and air.

pre-heaven qi. Eastern medicine term for energy (qi) that is inherited from our parents, analogous to genetic constitution in Western medicine.

prebiotics. The indigestible parts of some foods that are useful to beneficial microbes in the digestive tract.

preventive medicine. A medical specialty that focuses on the prevention of disease, not only in the individual patient but also in the community and population at large. A combination of clinical medicine and public health.

probiotics. Microbes that are ingested for their health benefits.

PubMed. A free search engine that can be used to find abstracts and articles on life sciences and biomedical subjects, maintained by the National Center for Biotechnology Information at the US National Library of Medicine.

qi. Eastern medicine term for the intelligent life force that flows through the body, often described in Western terms as "energy."

qigong. Mental, physical, and breathing exercises that cultivate qi. Related to taiji (see taiji).

short chain fatty acids. Beneficial fatty acids that contain less than six carbon atoms and are metabolized from indigestible fiber by colonic bacteria.

Silk Road. Ancient trading route between Asia and Europe that traversed Korea, China, India, Persia, and Europe.

Sun Si-Miao. Prolific seventh-century CE Chinese physician and herbalist who wrote two thirty-volume works on the practice of medicine. He was renowned for integrating Daoism with Buddhism and Confucianism and emphasized ethical behavior for physicians.

sympathetic nervous system. The division of the autonomic nervous system that prepares the body for intense physical activity, commonly referred to as the "fight or flight" response.

taiji. A Chinese martial art form, but also a series of slow, meditative movements that, when performed regularly, can improve health and well-being. Related to qigong (see qigong).

tui na. A method of Chinese bodywork or massage

ulcerative colitis. A type of inflammatory bowel disease (IBD) that can cause chronic inflammation and ulcers in the colon and rectum as well as manifestations in joints, skin, eyes, bones, kidneys, and liver.

vagus nerve. The longest nerve of the autonomic nervous system, largely responsible for conveying sensory input from the internal organs to the brain and relaying nerve impulses from the brain that increase the parasympathetic signals to internal organs, modulating their function; for example, lowering the heart rate and increasing the process of digestion.

World Health Organization (WHO). An agency of the United Nations, established in 1948, intended to improve international public health.

Wu Xing. Known in English as the Five Phases or Five Elements. The cosmological scheme that describes interactions among natural phenomena such as the changing of the seasons, developed in ancient China millennia ago and used in astrology, military strategy, and medicine.

yin-yang theory. The theory that states that all phenomena are composed of two opposite conditions or characteristics. These opposites cannot be separated; together, they represent the unified whole.

Index

About the Authors

Dr. Catherine Kurosu

Born, raised, and trained in Canada, Dr. Catherine Kurosu graduated from the University of Toronto School of Medicine in 1990. She completed her internship and residency at the same institution and qualified as a specialist in obstetrics and gynecology in 1995. Dr. Kurosu has studied and worked in Canada, the United States, Mexico, and Chile. Through her travels, she has learned that 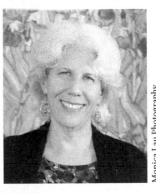 there are many ways to approach a problem and that the patient usually understands their illness best. By combining the patient's insight with medical guidance, effective treatment plans can be developed.

In 2006, Dr. Kurosu became a diplomate of the American Board of Holistic Medicine, now known as the American Board of Integrative Holistic Medicine. In 2009, she became certified as a medical acupuncturist through the David Geffen School of Medicine at UCLA and the Helms Medical Institute. Dr. Kurosu became a member of the American Academy of Medical Acupuncture, then a diplomate of the American Board of Medical Acupuncture, which confers this title on practitioners with increasing experience.

Since then, Dr. Kurosu has completed a master of science in Oriental medicine, graduating from the Institute of Clinical Acupuncture and Oriental Medicine in Honolulu. In 2015, she became a licensed acupuncturist and in 2018 a diplomate in Oriental medicine through the National Certification Commission for Acupuncture and Oriental Medicine.

Dr. Kurosu now lives on Oʻahu with her husband, Rob, and daughter, Hannah, where she practices integrative medicine, blending Western and Eastern approaches to patient care.

Dr. Aihan Kuhn

A graduate of Hunan Medical University in China (now called Xiangya Medical School) in 1982, Dr. Aihan Kuhn has focused her work on holistic healing since 1992. During many years of practice, she has accumulated much experience with holistic medicine and achieved a great reputation for her patient care and education work. Her patients benefit from her many important tips for self-improvement in their physical, emotional, and spiritual well-being, as well as from her simple and easy healing exercises to

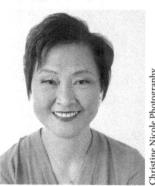

enable them to participate in their own healing. Dr. Kuhn incorporates taiji and qigong into her healing methodologies, changing the lives of those who have struggled for many years with no relief from conventional medicine. She offers many wellness programs, natural healing workshops, and professional training programs, such as taiji instructor training certification courses, qigong instructor training certification courses, and wellness tui na therapy certification courses. These highly rated programs have produced many quality teachers and therapists. Dr. Kuhn is president of the Taiji & Qi Gong Healing Institute (www.taichihealing.org), a nonprofit organization that promotes natural healing and prevention.

Dr. Kuhn lives with her husband, Gerry Kuhn, in Sarasota, Florida. For more information, please visit her website at www.draihankuhn.com.

Printed in the USA
CPSIA information can be obtained
at www.ICGtesting.com
JSHW012049140824
68134JS00035B/3348

9 781594 397455